AWAKENING THE SPINE

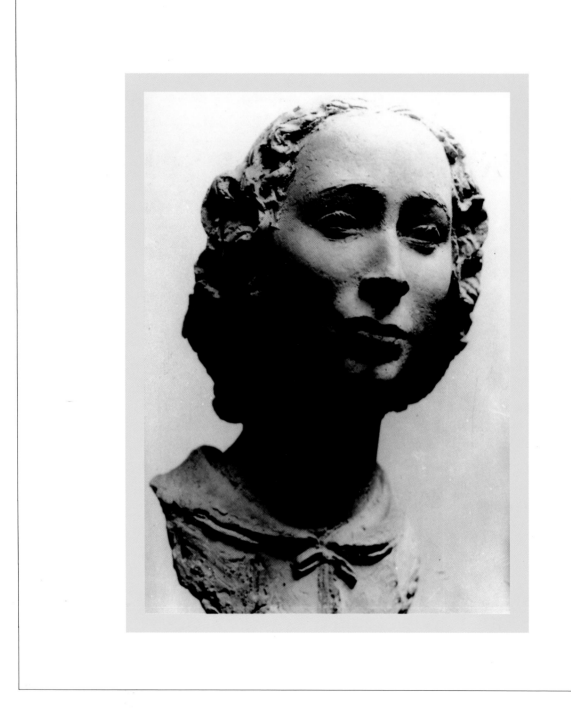

AWAKENING THE SPINE

The Stress-free New Yoga That Works with the
Body to Restore Health, Vitality and Energy

Vanda Scaravelli

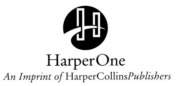

HarperOne
An Imprint of HarperCollins*Publishers*

HarperOne

HarperCollins books may be purchased for educational, business, or sales promotional use. For information please write: Special Markets Department, HarperCollins Publishers, 10 East 53rd Street, New York, NY 10022.

HarperCollins Web site: http://www.harpercollins.com

HarperCollins®, ☰®, and HarperOne™ are trademarks of HarperCollins Publishers.

Awakening the Spine was produced by Labyrinth Publishing (U.K.) Ltd.

Art direction and design by Magda Valine
Photography by Arturo Patten
Typesetting by The Word Shop, Bury, Britian

Library of Congress Cataloging-in-Publication Data

Scaravelli, Vanda.
Awakening the Spine : The Stress-free New Yoga That Work with the Body to Restore Health, Vatality and Energy / Vanda Scaravelli.
p. cm.
Includes index.
ISBN 978–0–06–250792–1
1. Yoga. Hatha. 2. Spine. I. Title.
RA781.7.S29   1991
613.7'046—dc20   90–85686

08 09 10 11 12 PE 20 19 18 17 16 15 14 13 12 11

C O N T E N T S

To B.K.S. Iyengar

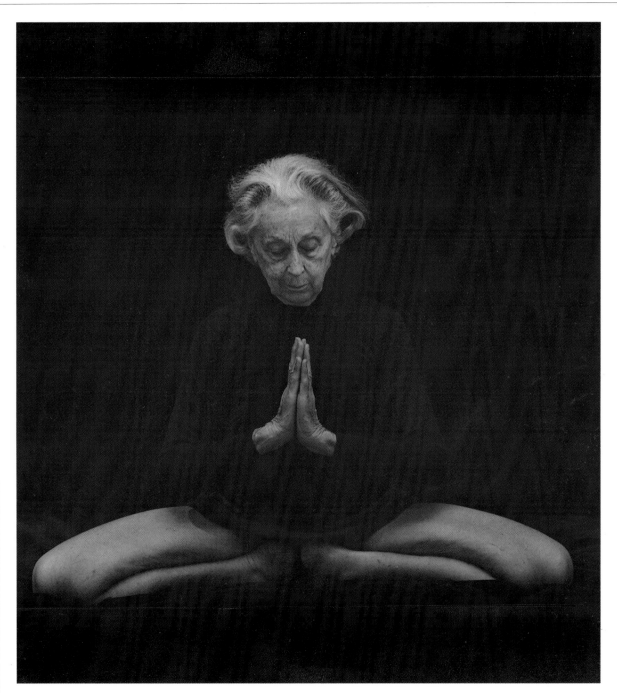

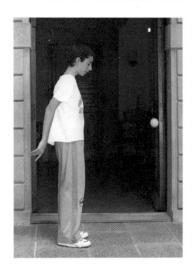

This page: The tennis ball bounces off the floor and falls again, pulled downwards by the force of gravity. *Right*: The Spiral galaxy in Coma Berenires.

Introduction

WHAT IS THIS NEW teaching? A revolution has to take place. A revolution based on one very simple physical truth. There is a division in the center of our back, where the spine moves simultaneously in two opposite directions: from the waist down towards the legs and the feet, which are pulled by gravity, and from the waist upwards, through the top of the head, lifting us up freely.

The pull of gravity under our feet makes it possible for us to extend the upper part of the spine, and this extension allows us also to release between the vertebrae. Gravity is like a magnet attracting us to the earth, but this attraction is not limited to pulling us down, it also allows us to stretch in the opposite direction towards the sky.

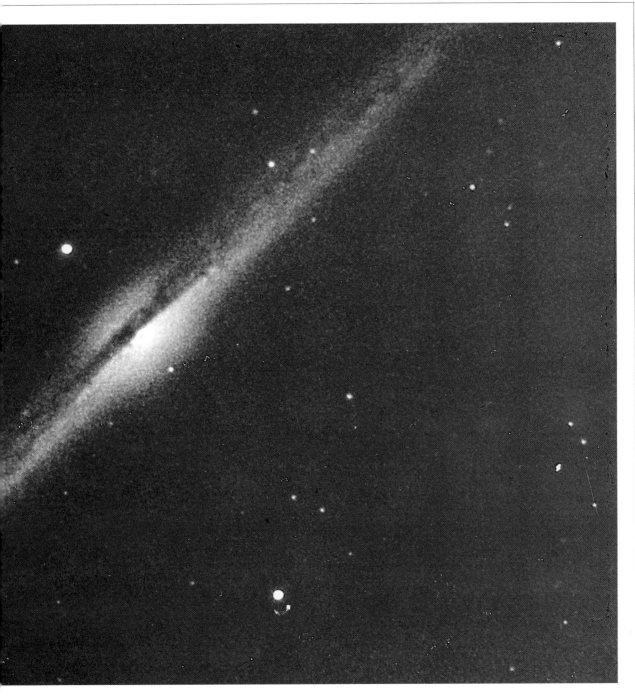

This is a natural process, ever-present not only in human beings but in all upright living things, in trees, in growing flowers and in plants. The roots of a tree are pulled deeply down towards the center of the earth while the trunk grows vertically towards the sky, elongating and spreading through the branches into the space around it. The deeper the roots penetrate into the ground, traveling below the surface of the earth, the taller and stronger grows the tree.

Above the surface of the earth the tree, mostly through its leaves, receives air, sun and rain water enabling it to develop its sap. Below the surface of the earth, by absorbing water and minerals through its roots, the tree receives nourishment and strength.

This central point of the tree, where it touches the earth's surface, corresponds in our body to the waist at the level of the fifth lumbar vertebra, where the human spine moves in both directions.

Goethe said that he could understand the falling of the apple (that gave Newton the idea of gravity) but he could not understand how a tree could grow in two opposite directions. This inexplicable cosmic interconnection of dynamic movements, following the law of gravity, is the same that moves the planets and holds the different worlds together.

Gravity attracts a planet and it is this very attraction which creates the lightness that gives it the ability to rotate in its spiral "revolution".

Each of the yoga poses is accompanied by breathing and it is during the process of exhalation that the spine can stretch and elongate without effort. We learn to elongate and extend, rather than to pull and push. Elongation and extension can only occur when the pulling and pushing has come to an end; this is the revolution.

For this revolution to occur, the muscles must not be activated through tension or effort but only through the much more powerful wave of extension, which is produced by gravity and breathing. We make use of the force of "anti-force", which gives us a new flow of energy – a sort of anti-gravity reflex, like the rebounding spring of a ball bouncing on the ground.

The resulting wave is extraordinarily powerful and helps us to find the right approach: an unexpected opening follows, an opening from within us, giving life to the spine, as though the body had to reverse and awaken into another dimension.

Right: The magnificence of the ramification of the tree is possible only because the roots grow deep within the earth, so that the trunk is strongly supported and can branch out wider and wider as the roots grow deeper and deeper with the years.

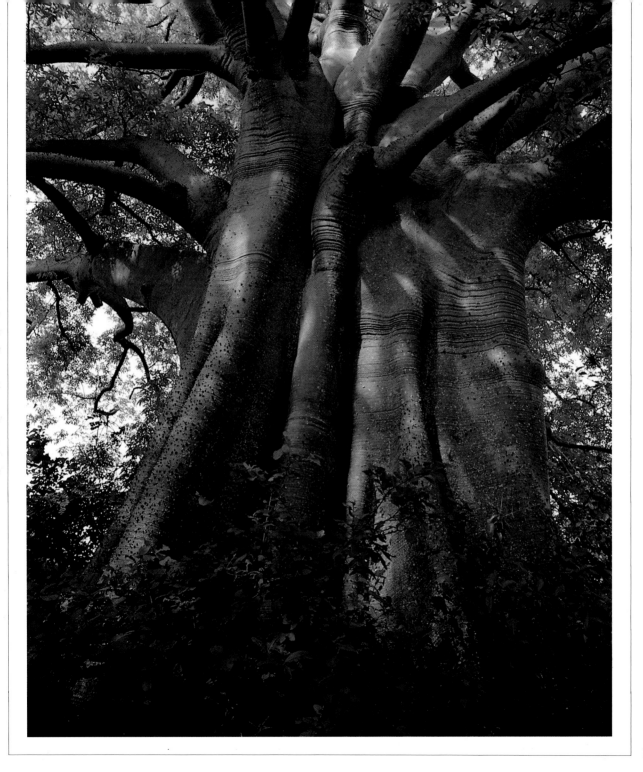

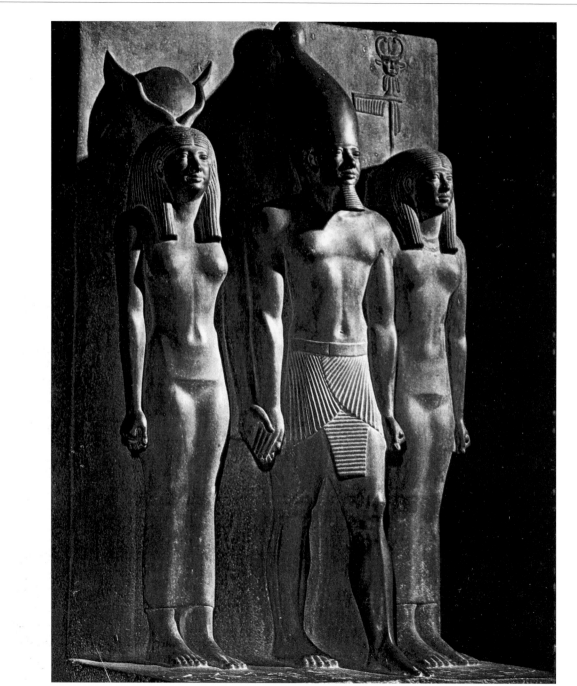

If we observe photographs of Egyptian statues we can see that the Egyptian spine was completely straight, adhering to the wall with no curve at the waist. The dignity of the Pharaohs is in their posture, for the complete elongation of the spine helps the body to regain its intended elegance.

The ancient Egyptians knew all about this. We can see it in their statues. This strength rises from their feet to the upper part of their bodies and an incredible energy explodes like fire from the heels to the top of the head. Hence they move with majesty, poise, and dignity.

The Pharaohs were Kings and Gods and therefore needed to discover something within their bodies that would make them great. This was the religion of the body.

The Egyptian spine was completely straight, adhering to the wall, as can be seen from the pictures in this book. There is no curve at the back of the waist. This is the very point where the spine opens and where the double movement takes place upwards and downwards at the same moment. If we look at the many different Egyptian statues, it is as though they wished to draw our attention to this one fact.

It seems that the artists who made these sculptures wanted to reveal and hide, at the same time, a mystery that was known only to initiates.

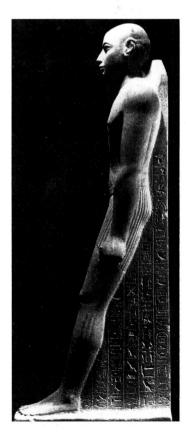

Looking closely at the pictures on these pages, it can be seen that Egyptians walked placing their heels down first with the knees straight, extending the soles from the heels to the toes. The soles of the feet and the palms of the hands are centers of vitality and by spreading, they also meet and receive energy from the earth.

Probably, the Egyptians did some kind of exercise that we could call yoga, but only in order to awaken the intelligence of the body which then, indirectly, made their minds sharper.

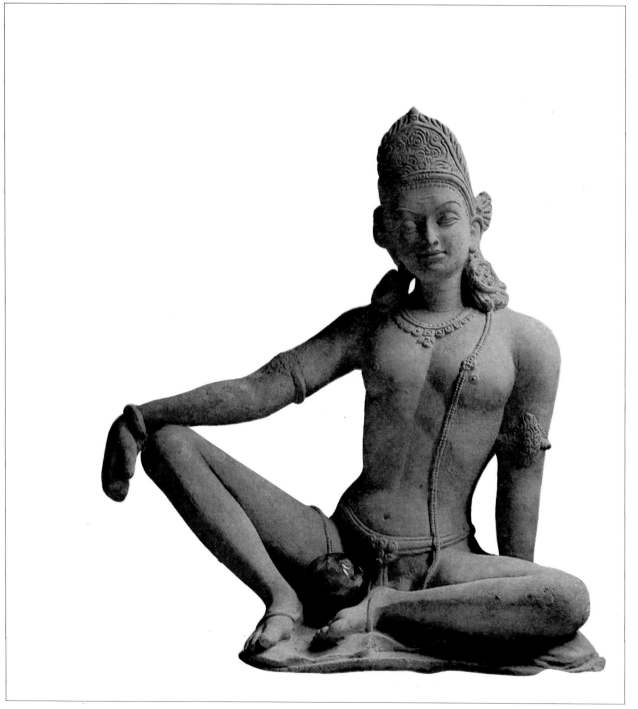

Part I

The Story of Stories

THE BOOK – HOW YOGA CAME TO ME – THE SONG OF THE BODY – GROWING TALLER DURING THE NIGHT – BEING YOUNG AGAIN – TRANSFORMATION – HOW TO RESPECT YOUR BODY – THE MIRACLE OF LIFE – ON TEACHING – REVERSING – GOING ROUND – WHAT DO WE MEAN BY RELAXATION? – HOW TO PRACTICE – NERVES – WHY ARE WE DOING YOGA? – ON TIME – MATTER AND ENERGY – THE IMPORTANCE OF DAILY PRACTICE – THE HEEL IN GREEK MYTHOLOGY – ON MEMORY AND AGE – MEETING OF BODY AND MIND – ON BEAUTY – THE FOOT IN THE CHINESE TRADITION – THE FOOT IN THE JAPANESE TRADITION – MOVEMENTS, THE ANCIENT TRADITION – THE FOOT IN THE INDIAN TRADITION – ON ATTENTION – ABOUT ORGANISATIONS – GRAVITY – THE EAGLE – ON WALKING – THE BRAIN – A MEETING WITH DEATH – THE NECESSITY OF AN EMPTY MIND – PRACTICAL ADVICE – THE ADVANTAGES OF DOING YOGA

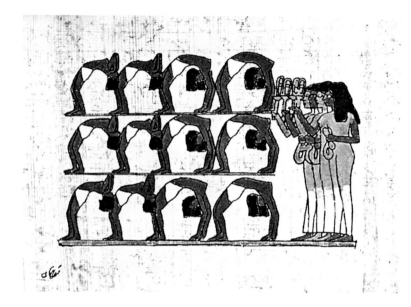

The Book

THIS IS NOT REALLY a yoga book nor a book on yoga, for yoga has been written about so much in recent years. It has become fashionable and people like to do it and talk about it. What we will try to do in this book is to create a much more serious approach towards our bodies, which have been neglected for so many years. This approach and attitude with regard to the body and the mind are absolutely different, and sometimes even opposite, from the casual way in which it has been done until now. You have to learn how to listen to your body, going with it and not against it, avoiding all effort or strain and centering your attention on that very delicate point, the back of the waist (where the spine moves in two opposite directions). You will be amazed to discover that, if you are kind to your body, it will respond in an incredible way.

Above: In this interesting Egyptian wall-painting we can see dancers preparing and performing Urdhva Dhanurāsana, or back-bend from standing. Possibly, the ancient Egyptians did some kind of exercise that we may call yoga. *Top right and bottom right:* In these wall-carvings again we can see the emphasis placed upon the feet in these posture that, like in yoga, work all the time to give roots and to support the body.

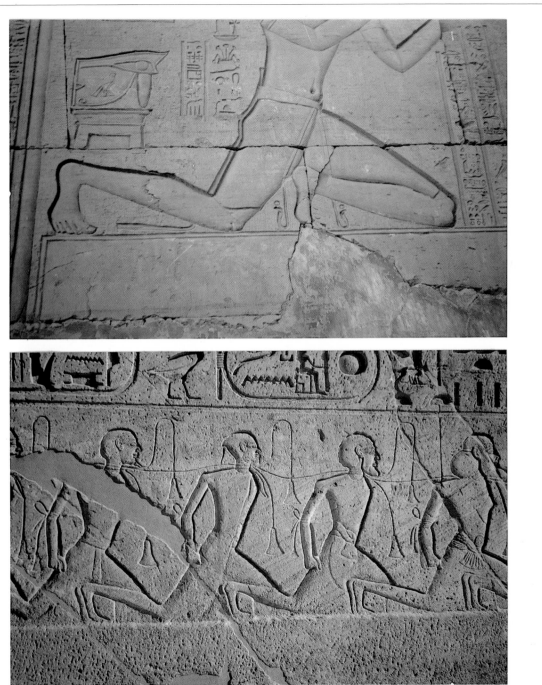

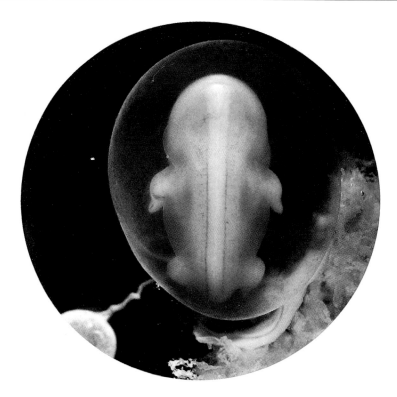

The first structure that is formed in the child's body (while still in the mother's womb) is the spine, and consequently all the other limbs, the arms, legs and hips, derive from it. For this reason the spine is of the greatest importance. If the movements you do during the day originate from the spine, then the action is correct. But to do this and feel the result of it takes some time.

The quadruped animals elongate their spines with each step. We should do the same while walking or standing; with two legs this is evidently more difficult, but, after all, it is only a question of stretching our knees from the heels, keeping the heels in contact with the ground.

Baby's spines are extremely soft and light and remain so for a very long time. Instead the adult spine is rigid and heavy and yoga, as intended here, consists in breaking bad habits and in re-educating the spine so as to bring back its original suppleness.

This is what is meant by the title of the book.

Above: The spinal cord from which the rest of the skeleton spreads is the first structure to be formed in the human embryo in the first weeks of life in the womb. The spine is a delicate and yet extremely important axis that supports the whole body. Thick blood vessels, the vertebral arteries, run down either side of the spinal cord.

How Yoga Came to Me

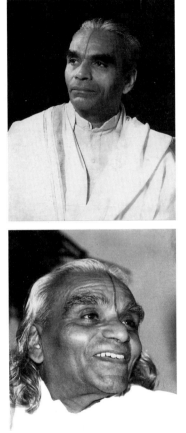

I AM OFTEN ASKED HOW I started yoga. I learned yoga from B.K.S. Iyengar* in Gstaad, Switzerland. He came from India, invited by the well known violinist Yehudi Menuhin. During the summer months J.Krishnamurti* was our guest at Chalet Tannegg and Iyengar gave him yoga lessons every morning from seven to eight. Iyengar was so kind as to give me a lesson each day as well. I was fortunate enough to have private lessons from him for many years thereafter.

I trusted Mr. Iyengar completely, aware of the privilege of being able to work with him. My body offered no resistance, like clay in his hands, and he could do what he wanted with it. During those years my health improved and I felt much better. I am really grateful for all he did for me and for those wonderful yoga lessons.

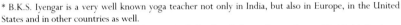

* B.K.S. Iyengar is a very well known yoga teacher not only in India, but also in Europe, in the United States and in other countries as well.
He lives in Poona, in the state of Maharastra in India. People from all over the world visit his Institute, the "Ramamani Iyengar Memorial Institute." Ramamani was the name of his late wife. His son and daughter help him with his work as the number of his students increases every day.
His numerous pupils have created many centers where his teaching is largely spreading.
His book, "Light on Yoga", has become popular among those who want to practice seriously and is of great help to them.
Iyengar has the rare gift of being able to communicate his enthusiasm and thoroughness of knowledge on the subject of yoga to his pupils. We can say that he has the genius of teaching, having the possibility to act with his willpower on the body of others, taking it "psychologically" into his hands, as if it was his own, to bring it to the point he wants.
He is now 72 years old, still in perfect shape, travels everywhere and his practice is growing every day.

* Born near Madras, Jiddu Krishnamurti (1895–1986) was fourteen when he was taken under the guardianship of Mrs Annie Besant, socialist, reformer and President of the International Theosophical Society at Adyar, near Madras. She and her colleague, C.W. Leadbeater, believed that Krishnamurti was the vehicle for the Messiah whose coming the Theososphists had predicted. The Order of the Star in the east, an organisation dedicated to preparing mankind for the coming of the World Teacher, was formed in 1911 with Krishnamurti at its head. In the same year he was brought to England to be privately educated and trained for his role. In 1929, however, he shocked the world with a dramatic public disavowel of his role and declared that he did not want disciples.
Long recognised as one of the world's foremost spiritual teachers, Kirshnamurti dedicated his life to speaking throughout the world, giving public talks and private interviews. His philosophy has attracted such figures as Nehru, Bernard Shaw, Aldous Huxley and the Dalai Lama. Over the years his annual gatherings in India, at Ojai, California, at Saanen in Switzerland and at Brockwood Park in Hampshire attracted thousands of people of different nationality. Krishnamurti also wrote many books among which are "The Impossible Question", "Beyond Violence" and "The Wholeness of Life".

Portraits of B.K.S. Iyengar, a master of yoga, who was invited to come to Gstaad, Switzerland, by the well-known violinist Yehudi Menuhin. Mr. Iyengar taught the author yoga every morning during the numerous summer months that he visited Chalet Tannegg.

Later on, when I met Desicachar (another exceptional yoga teacher)*, invited by Jiddu Krishnamurti, I understood the importance of breathing.

Desicachar's father Krishnamacharya (teacher and brother in law of Mr. Iyengar)* could stop his heart beating. This was testified to by several doctors, among them a friend of ours named Prof. Marcault*, who went to India with a doctor. They were able to take a cardiogram of his heart in which one could see the heart beats slowly diminishing and, after stopping for a few seconds, starting to beat again.

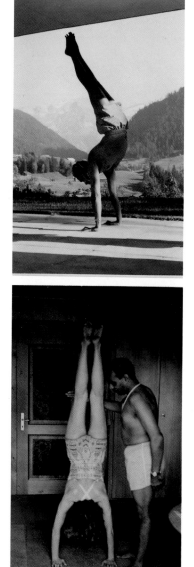

* Desicachar is a serious, profound and special yoga teacher as well as an agreeable person to be with, one can laugh and have fun with him.
He left his promising engineering career to continue the training and teaching of yoga, which he inherited from his father, Krishnamacharya who was highly esteemed not only in the yoga field, but also for his knowledge of the Sanskrit language and religious scriptures.
Krishnamacharya went into the Himalaya retreats where he had the privilege of being instructed by the Masters who have lived there from the beginning of time. He wished to remain with them but was sent back to transmit to the world the teaching he had received. Desicachar lives in Madras where he created the "Krishnamacharya Yoga Mandir" – an institution recognised by the "Health and Family Welfare Department" of the Government of Tamil Nadu.
A group of European students bring forward his teaching under the name of "Vini Yoga", which means to adapt the teaching of Yoga to each individual.
In his book "Religiousness in Yoga", translated in many languages, the connection of breathing with the āsanas is carefully explained.

* Professor Emile Marcault came from Montpellier in France with his family to teach French Literature at the University of Pisa, in Italy. Later on he became President of the French Theosophical Society.
He lectured in three languages: French, English and Italian. As well as being erudite in ancient Greek and Latin, his culture embraced both fields of literature and science with wide knowledge of subjects such as Physics, Astronomy, Astrology and Psychology.
He was asked by Count Visconti di Modrone to join him in Milan and to work in his pharmaceutical company "Carlo Erba di Milano" to sustain his employees and talk with their families, giving them psychological advice and moral help. This happened at a time when little attention was paid to the welfare of the working class.
Pushed by an insatiable fever to understand the roots of humanity, Prof. Marcault decided to tour India with Prof. La Brosse in order to learn more about the control of the body. Together they visited many so-called Gurus.
They investigated the exceptional abilities that these extraordinary men possessed and with which they were capable of reversing the functions of the body. Some of them were not easy to contact as they lived aloof in remote places and only wanted to show their capacities to seriously interested people.

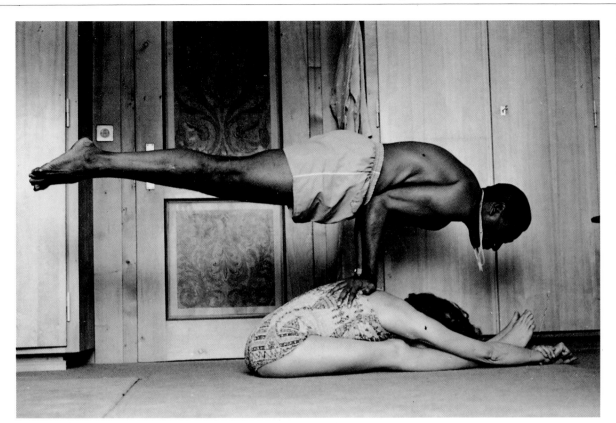

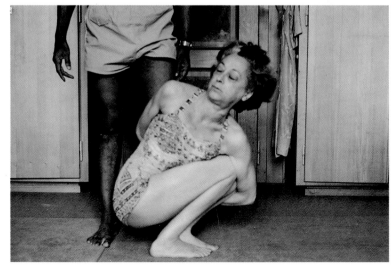

B.K.S. Iyengar teaching the author the Asanas. *Above:* Paschimottanāsana and below the teacher helps the pupil with one of the twists.

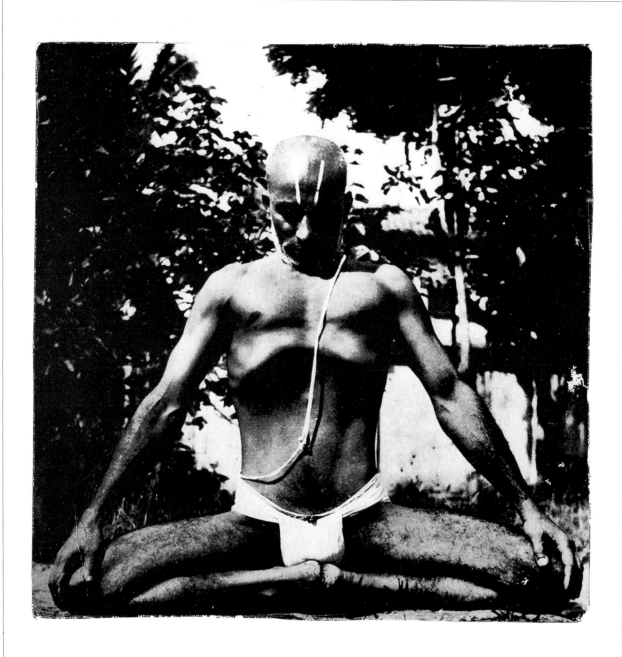

The heart is the most important organ in our body and it can be controlled by long training in breathing exercises. It is not possible to teach how to breathe, but by watching and listening to the beating of the heart and the movements of the lungs, following attentively the inhalations and exhalations, one can discover a great deal.

To follow the way the spine functions during this process of breathing is of the greatest interest. The wave of expansion while exhaling, originating from the spine, is the basis of our teaching.

I continued to have lessons with Desicachar for several years, when he came each summer to our chalet at Gstaad, Switzerland, to teach Krishnamurti. He liked to drive and said to a friend of mine that he was a little scared when I drove too fast! But Italians like speed! From him, I learned that one cannot disassociate the positions (āsanas) from breathing, they are inter-related and it is not possible to conceive any āsana pose without connecting it with breathing.

One often sees students holding their breath while performing a difficult pose. This is counter-productive and fundamentally wrong because it blocks the lovely movement, while the expansion of the lungs in connection with the spine is in action.

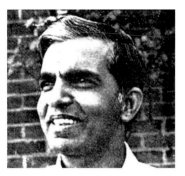

Opposite: Krishnamacharya breathing in Mulabandhāsana. The abdomen and the stomach is completely drawn in, leaving, in the upper part of the lungs, a space between the base of the rib cage and the lower abdomen. *Top right*: A portrait of Desicachar, Krishnamacharya's son. This remarkable man taught the author the importance of breathing correctly. *Bottom left*: A human heart, showing arteries and veins that supply blood to the cardiac muscles. The heart can be controlled by long training in breathing exercises. *Bottom right*: False-color X-ray of normal human lungs, showing the heart as a white, pear-shaped form. With inhalation and exhalation, the lungs move like a sponge squeezed in one's hands. A long exhalation enables even the smallest of the alveoli to be cleansed and renewed with oxygenation.

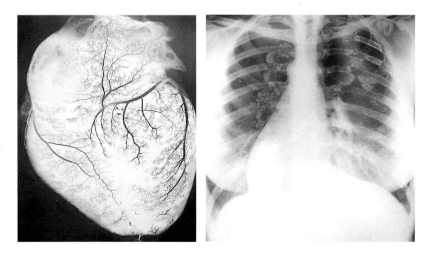

23

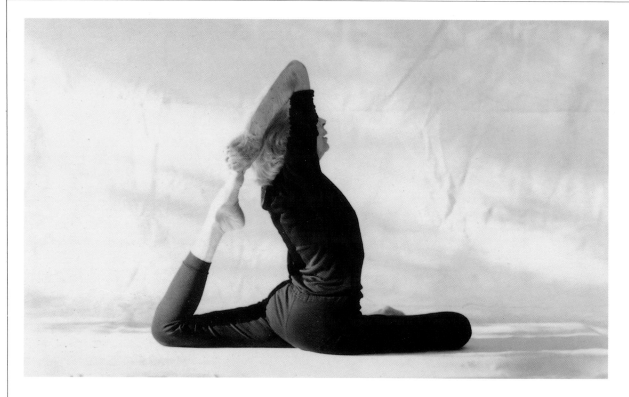

But it was only when I remained alone that I discovered a new world in this field, a world without aim and without competition, where the body can start again to function naturally and happily, allowing expansion to take place in space.

Iyengar and Desicachar were no longer coming to Gstaad, therefore I was stimulated to find a different approach that would permit those who were around me to continue their practice without becoming exhausted.

Gravity seemed to be the answer and from there started a new way of doing the āsanas.

It is not so much the performance of the exercises that matters, but rather the way we are doing them.

We have three friends: gravity, breath, and wave (connected with the supple movement of extension along the spine). These three companions (fused in one) should be constantly with us.

Above: Ekapada Rajakapotanasana. *Opposite:* painting of an Egyptian dancer performing a pose very similar to a yogic asana. When the mind understands the movement, the body follows and is happy to extend and elongate with freedom, like in a dance.

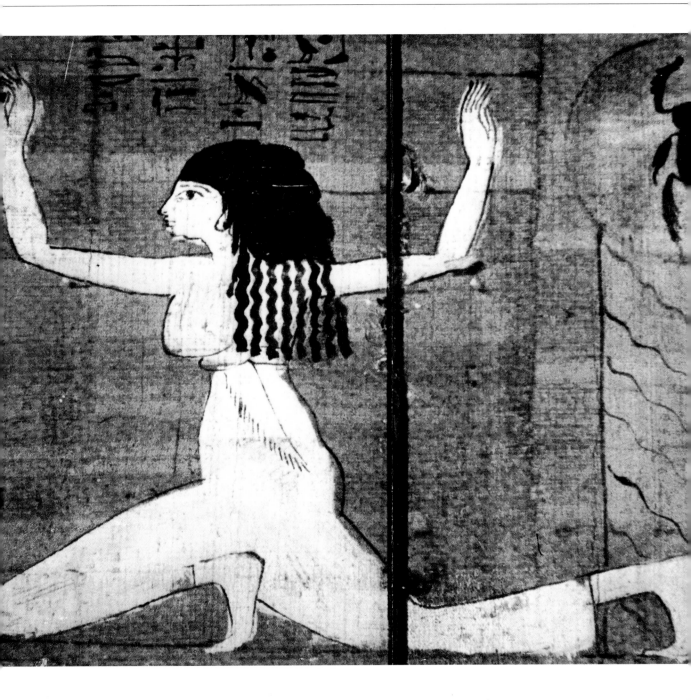

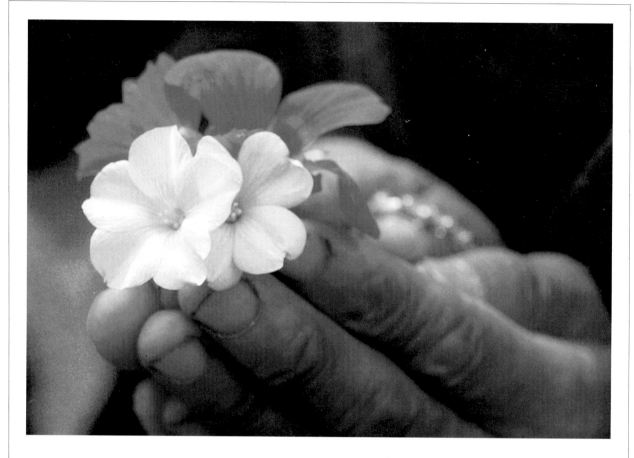

Gautama the Buddha once arrived to give his morning discourse to a huge gathering of followers. But he sat in silence holding a flower. Mahakasyapa, his oldest disciple suddenly laughed, upon which the Buddha declared "The most precious treasure I can now hand to you" and gave him the flower. This is a traditional example of a transmission beyond words – the greatest form of teaching possible.

Some may ask why I write on a subject where we can only really achieve a result through training and example. But in this teaching there are no achievements and no results. It consists simply in the cleansing and revival of the body and the reawakening of the spine. This purification will give us health and a chance of healing whatever may not be right with the body.

It is also a joy to share something one likes with others. I have seen so many people damage themselves by doing poses in the wrong way. This is why, after much hesitation, I decided to communicate my experiences, and even if only one or two people should benefit by a clearer picture, it will be enough.

From the act of observation in which attention is awakened, arises the art of teaching. The art of teaching is clarity and the art of

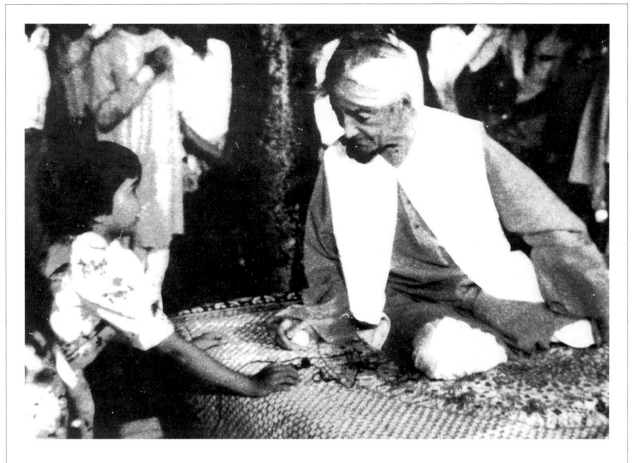

Krishnamurti talking to a child.

learning is to listen. All my pupils teach. It is imperative to communicate to others what you see and feel. To teach is an urge and a necessity. When you see someone in a cage or in a dark room, you cannot help but open the door of the prison.

There is so much joy in teaching what you feel is right. This changed perception will give you wings to find the best words and adequate expressions to transmit to your pupils what you have seen with your mind.

Never doubt. It is always possible for the body to carry out whatever has been projected with exactitude by the mind. If the logic and evidence of what you say is accepted by the brain, the body follows it. "The seeing is the doing", as Krishnamurti often repeated.

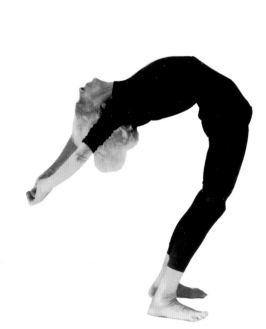

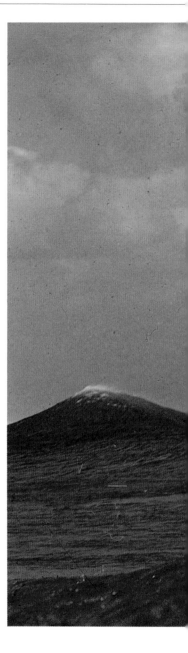

The Song of the Body

THERE IS A WAY OF DOING yoga poses that we call "āsanas", without the slightest effort. Movement is the song of the body. Yes, the body has its own song from which the movement of dancing arises spontaneously. In other words, the liberation of the upper part of the body (the head, neck, arms, shoulders, and trunk) produced by the acceptance of gravity in the lower part of the body (legs, feet, knees, and hips) is the origin of lightness, and dancing is its expression. This song, if you care to listen to it, is beauty. We could say that it is part of nature. We sing when we are happy and the body goes with it like waves in the sea.

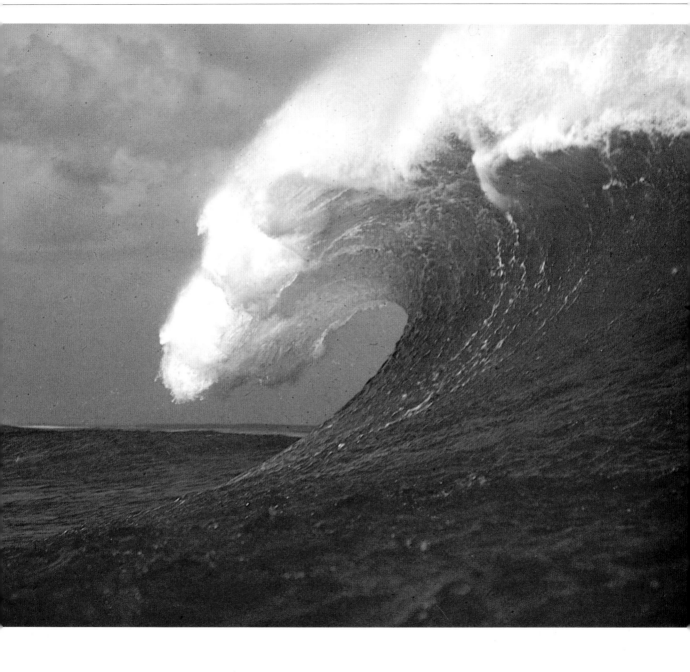

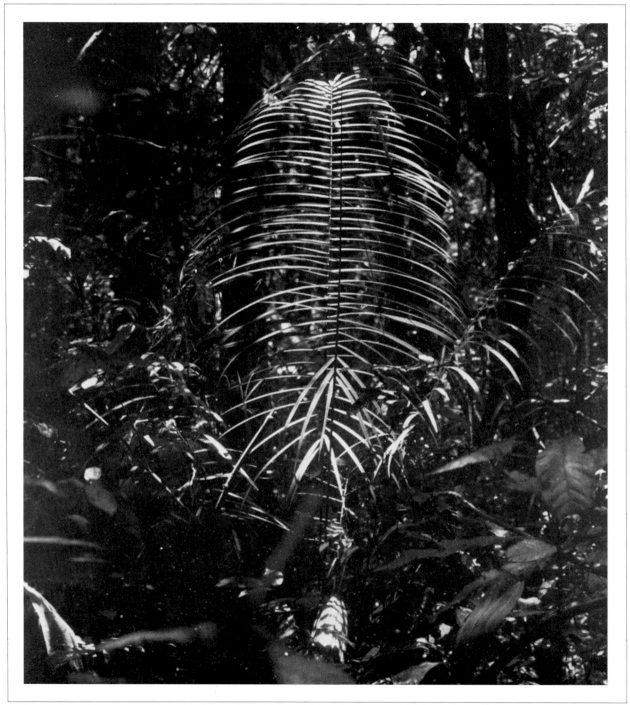

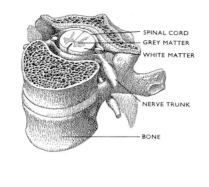

In this position of the spine we can clearly distinguish the disks that enable the vertebrae to move forwards and backwards and to rotate. Without them all movement would be impossible.

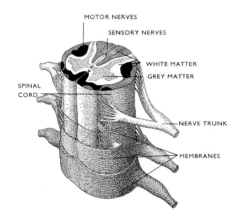

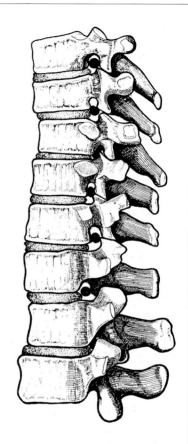

Growing Taller During the Night

ALREADY IN 1935, the hydrophobic property of cartilage had been demonstrated. It is a well-known fact that "we are all shorter at night by three-quarters of an inch, resulting from the total cartilage compression during the day. This is the reason why most drivers tend to adjust their rear view mirrors at the end of the day".

It was also noted that "all cartilage as well as the intervertebral disc, also imbibe water during rest in the horizontal position". [1]

The relief of pressure on the cartilage can be maintained also during the day by performing spinal extensions.

The human spine is capable of growing in both directions just like a plant. At the end of the day, most people are shorter than in the morning due to the cartilage compression during the day. The Asanas help to extend the space between the vertebrae, relieving thus the stress to the spinal cord accumulated during the day's activities.

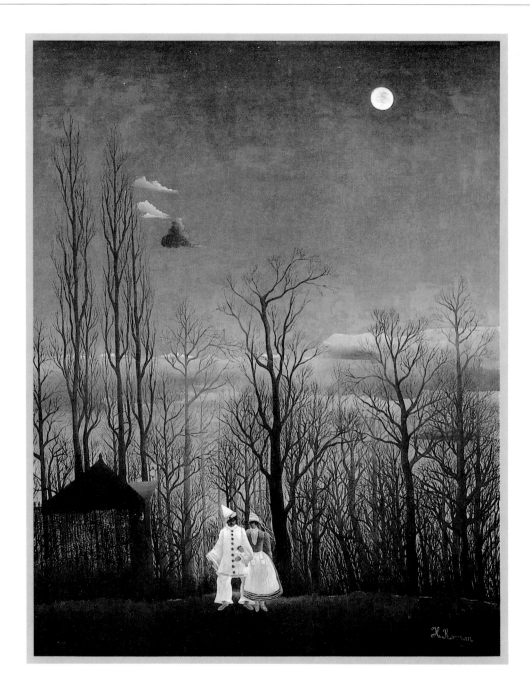

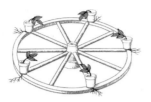

Being Young Again

THE FUNCTION OF THE BODY is to collect energy from the ground. By grasping the gravity of the earth we become connected to the soil, from which also plants and trees receive their nourishment (the other part is given by air, water and the sun).

This contact with the soil will enable us to expand not only vertically but also on a horizontal level all around (like the branches of a tree), extending and bending forwards, sideways and backwards.

The function of the spine is to elongate, and in this elongation its elasticity and youth are regained. It is not a battle against old age, but rather a bringing back to life of those parts in the body that have been neglected for so long and have lost their suppleness.

We have lost contact with our bodies, and re-establishing this connection is what we try to do. The body should respond immediately to the requests of the mind. The less the gap between the two, the more efficient the action will be (in medical terms this is called "reflex").

There is no age limit, one can start yoga when 70 or 80 years old and no damage will occur if the movements originate from the spine. People feel elated and it gives them comfort and encouragement to discover that it is possible for them to control and modify their bodies. To talk about old age as an impediment is an excuse to be lazy. A lady of 70 was delighted to follow the movement along her back saying, "*It feels like being young again*".

Above: These two drawings represent a plant's response to gravity. When a seedling is grown inside a tube, its stem will turn upwards and its roots downwards as soon as they escape the tube's restricting walls. This reaction, positive for root and negative for stem, is known as geotropism – a response to gravity. The English experimenter, Thomas Knight, proved this more than 150 years ago. He fixed plants on a revolving wheel so that the centrifugal force counteracted gravity. The roots then grow outwards and the stems inwards, exactly as if gravity had been acting horizontally. *Opposite:* To dance, to move freely, incites a positive response in the body and causes an increase of energy.

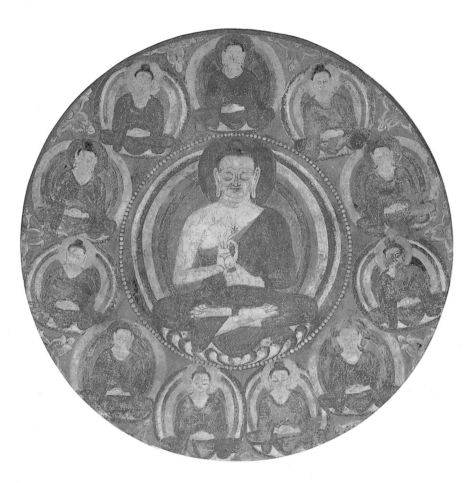

Transformation

READING THESE DESCRIPTIONS is like putting food on a tray but to get the flavor and taste of it, you have to eat it. The food is agreeable and easy to digest. Teachers enjoy teaching and this makes it easy for pupils to learn. This new attitude in performing yoga āsanas is like an initiation. To absorb the teaching requires infinite time and no ambition, but as teachers like to teach it thus becomes easy for the pupils to learn.

Above: Indian image depicting all the aspects of Buddhahood.
Opposite: A Buddhist devotee paying homage to the sacred feet of the Buddha.

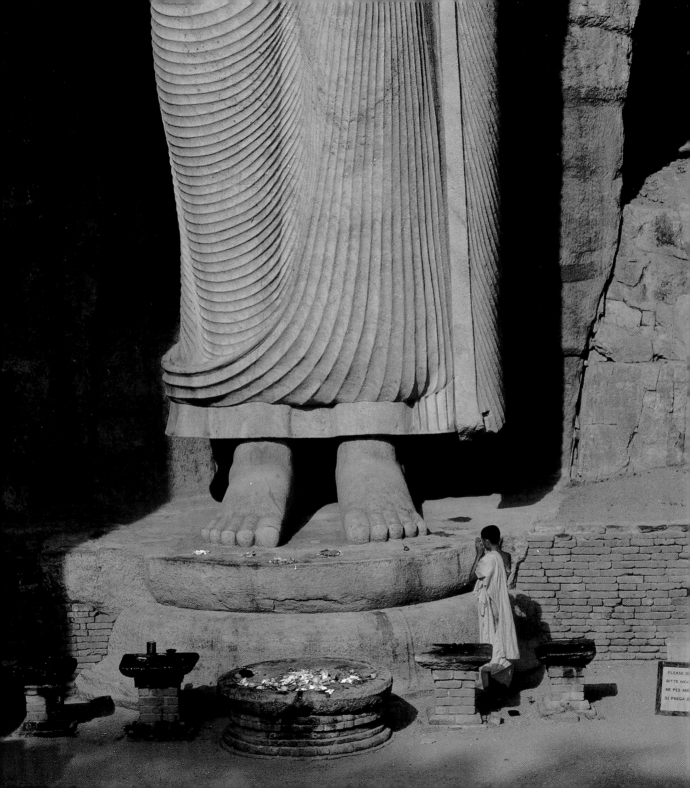

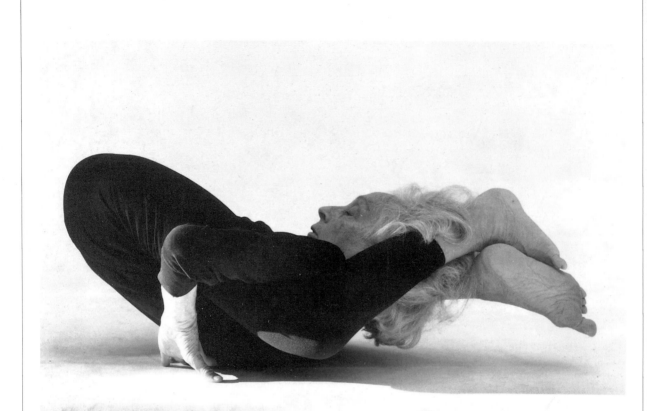

Practice transforms us. We need to eat less, because we assimilate more and therefore there is a loss of unnecessary weight. We become more beautiful, our faces change and our walk gains in elasticity. Our way of standing is steady and poised, our legs are firmer, and our toes and feet spread out, giving us more stability. Our chests expand, the muscles of the abdomen start to work, the head is lighter on the neck (like the corolla of a flower on its stem moving easily with flexibility while the wind blows). To watch these enchanting changes is amazing.

A different life begins and the body expresses a happiness never felt before. These are not just words; it actually happens.

Above: Yoga Nidrāsana, the yoga sleeping pose. Practice transforms the body and the mind and a new life begins.

Opposite: A triumphant trumpeter swan displaying its beauty and freedom. It is important that the body regains its natural joy of movement in order that a total, physical transformation may occur.

36

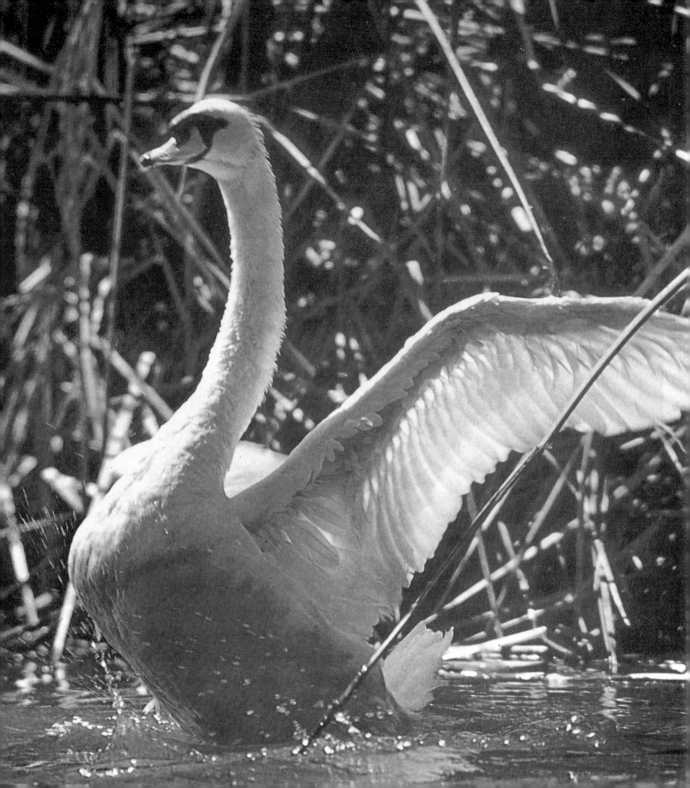

How to Respect your Body

THE WAY WE LIVE IS DESTRUCTIVE to the body; there is no respect towards its needs and demands. We destroy, little by little, that precious, complex, vital, vessel of life we received at birth, why? For ambition? For a final cause? For the sake of our children, or of our family, for the "superior" mind, the "higher" self, the glorification of the brain, enlightenment, etc.?

All religions encourage self-sacrifice, but when we are ill we pray to God to heal us. How inconsistent we are! To be simple, to appreciate what has been given to us, and to take care of our body, is an act of humility. A group of people after a seminar, asked me about death. To die is alright, we all have to die sooner or later, but what we must do is not allow the body to degenerate while living. By doing yoga in the proper way, we should be able to maintain its purity until the end.

Do not fight your body. Do not carry the world on your shoulders like Atlas. Drop that heavy load of unnecessary baggage and you will feel better.

Do not kill the instinct of the body for the glory of the pose. Do not look at your body like a stranger, but adopt a friendly approach towards it. Watch it, listen to it, observe its needs, its requests, and even have fun. Play with it as children do, sometimes it becomes very alert and swift.

To be sensitive is to be alive.

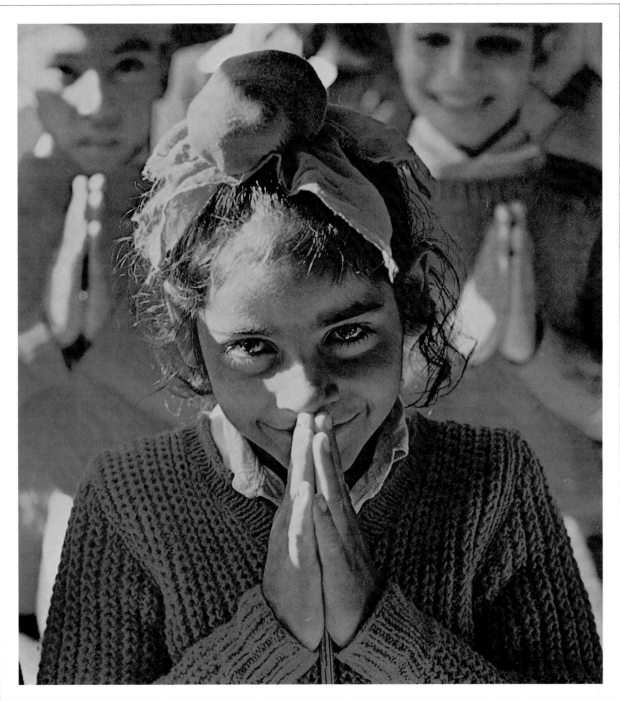

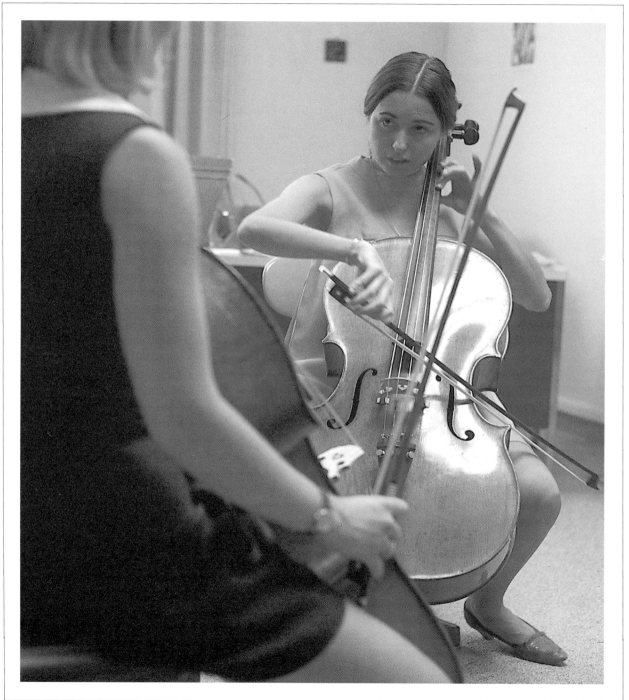

When some difficulty arises we can always find a different movement, since the body is surprisingly able to adjust itself. It has its own intelligence and is willing to cooperate in finding a solution to any problem. One has only to approach problems with patience, care and attention.

Nobody can help you to do this. "*You have to become your own teacher and your own disciple*" (these are Krishnamurti's words).

People have all kinds of misconceptions about yoga. One must not think that the exercises are going to give us a higher perspective in a mystical or spiritual direction. They are simply refreshing the body, like a shower, cleansing us from the dirt and impurities accumulated during the day. It is like tuning an instrument before playing it. The movements are healthy and we receive physical advantages from doing them. Arms and legs need motion and any form of activity is good for us, such as walking, running, aerobics, golf, martial arts, gymnastics, or other forms of physical training. But our sports have become competitive and man spoils them through his insatiability for glory and success. Even the arts have become a means of self-affirmation.

Yoga has nothing to do with acrobatics or spectacular exhibitionism, even though some poses rather look like it. Students are sometimes inclined to force the flexibility of their bodies to the maximum, but this leads nowhere.

Yoga goes much deeper. Sometimes unexpected things happen that cannot be easily explained, like healings, bursts of crying, and other similar discharges of pressure. When tensions leave, the body goes back to its original state, and balance is re-established.

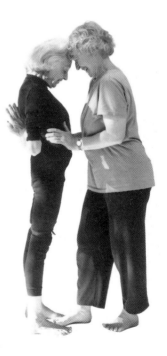

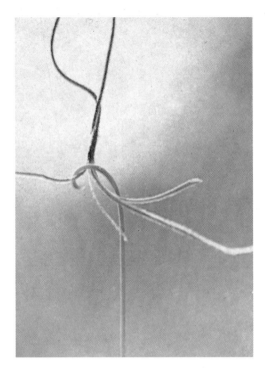

The Miracle of Life

THE BODY HAS ITS OWN WAY of fighting illness, readjusting itself to harmony.

Man wants to survive and be well and will find infinite ways to serve his necessities. There are no obstacles to this tremendous urge to live. The body will always discover a way to overcome the difficulties that are an impediment to its existence. To live is one of the greatest miracles.

The force of life in nature is so astonishingly strong. One asks how it is possible for a plant, a blade of grass, to grow in a street squeezed and suffocated by heavy asphalt, and still find its contact with the soil through a tiny little hole from where it meets the earth. And it lives!

On the stone battlements of our country house there grows a cypress tree that even has a few berries on it. We have never been able to understand how it could get its nourishment. It is a mystery!

Above: A species of Spanish moss anchors a green smilax tendril. In order to reach the light in the shadier recesses of a forest, plants grow in a variety of unexpected forms, including two species "helping" each other for the one common purpose. *Opposite:* A fig tree blossoms out of a hard rock. The force of life in nature is astonishingly strong.

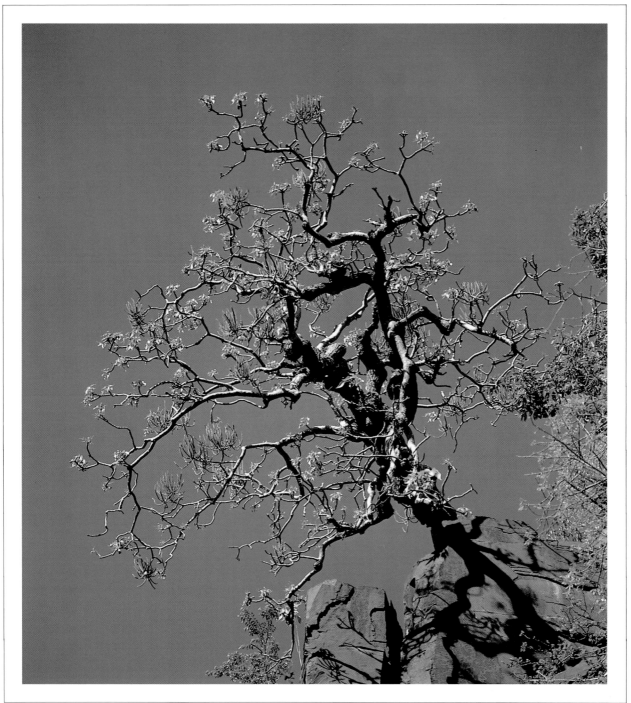

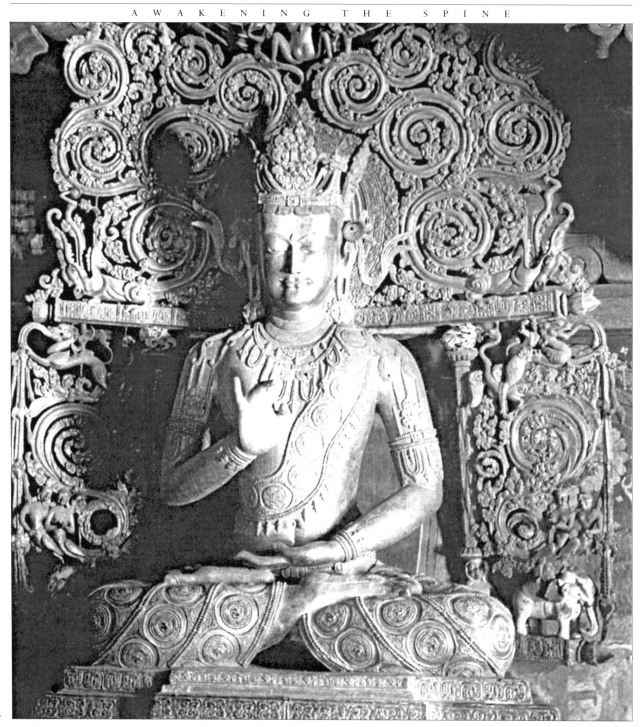

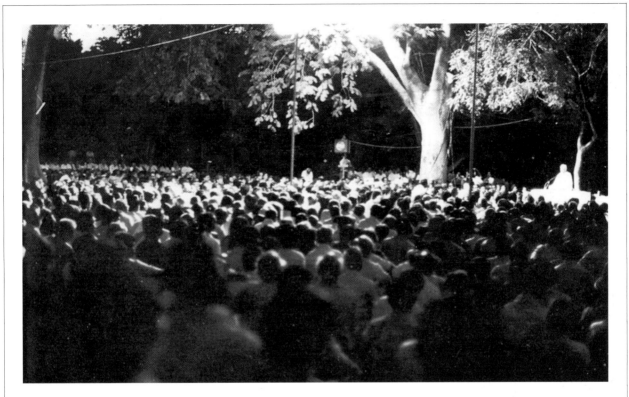

On Teaching

TEACHING IS THE HIGHEST LEVEL of work required by civilization in the world. To show the importance of teaching in his country, Krishnamurti used to tell us how in ancient Indian tradition, the teacher was placed at the very summit of the hierarchy. Even the King consulted teachers for their advice.

The lowest caste was that of the "Sudra". They could do whatever they wished, nothing was required from them.

Then came the "merchants". They made money from commerce and were allowed to eat, drink, have sexual relationships, and live the way they wanted.

Next came the military caste, the "warriors". They had a strict code of behavior. They had their own discipline, their own laws. They had to obey their own rules. (This caste included the Kings).

Above: Krishnamurti's last talk in Vasant Vihar, Adyar, Madras. January 3rd 1986
Left: Amoghasiddhi, one of the five manifestations of the Buddha. *The Kyangphu Monastery*.

The King's duties had to be strictly respected. He had to live in the greatest austerity, marry the right woman, have children only in certain periods of the year (in keeping with the ascendant or ascending phases of the moon, according to his religion). His life was in the hands of the teachers.

Above all the castes were the "Gurus", the "teachers". Kings and ministers consulted them on how to organize their lives. It was the Gurus who decided and directed their actions, and through their wisdom told them what to do and how to behave in different circumstances. They were therefore also responsible for the people and for their country.

This is no longer the case in India today, but it gives an idea of the position held by the teachers in the past.

To teach is an act of love. To teach yoga is also a responsibility, because occasionally certain centers are awakened in which the energy released can be tremendously powerful. This energy is not meant to be used for personal or egoistic purposes, but for other people's sake. To teach implies also a certain vigilance and dedication in everyday life.

This is why, in the past, this practice was limited to the very few.

There are no good pupils, there are only good teachers. Teaching is not an imposition of the teacher's will over that of the pupil, not at all. Teaching starts with freedom and ends with freedom.

A receptive state is required on the part of the pupil, a feeling of acceptance, even before the brain sees the truth of what is shown; an empty free space that one might call "innocence". It is from here that intelligence starts to function. The aim of the teacher is to awaken interest and curiosity in the mind of the pupil, giving him a clear picture of the subject. His explanations should be so evident and logical that the pupil cannot but grasp the significance of what is said.

Understanding leads to independence and to freedom.

Right: Portrait of Appa Sahib. This small child, eyes blackened with kohl, was a descendant of the noblest Maratha house in Maharastra, a region near Bombay.

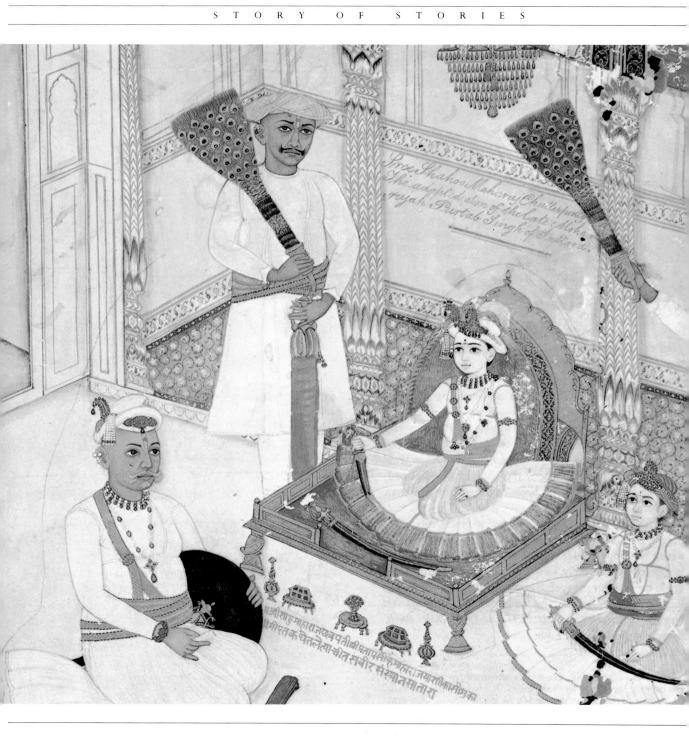

Reversing

WE USUALLY LIVE ON THE FRONT part of our bodies and we have developed more on that part, where most of our sensory organs are situated: eyes, nose, mouth, shoulders, hands and chest.

Now we have to reverse our attention giving consideration to the back of our body.

EYES.   We should be able to look from the back of the head, following the channel that reaches the skull. This will not only give us a wider and enlarged field of vision and a better perspective where the sides will be included, but our eyes will also be able to rest and gain benefit.

CEREBELLUM.   When you relax the cerebellum, you will feel how it extends from one ear to the other, unfolding, like a leaf, at the back of the brain.

NECK.   The neck, in line with the spine, follows the shape of the shoulders, keeping the head and chin in place, as the new pull is felt along the back.

LUNGS.   The lungs work and function only at their upper level, and the breath never reaches their lowest part, where they narrow down. That very last section is difficult to penetrate, as we are not accustomed to inhale so deeply.

HIPS.   By activating the hips at the base of our back, the weight of the body is going to sink down heavily. Let it drop, as if you were getting rid of a sack of potatoes. From the waist upwards the movement is the opposite, giving freedom to the upper part of the body and thereby increasing the opening and expansion of the lungs which will give greater potentiality to the breathing.

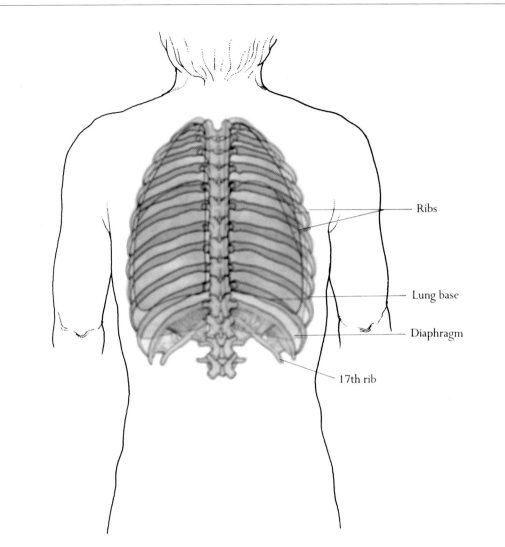

Ribs

Lung base

Diaphragm

17th rib

KNEES.   The back of the legs (especially the back of the knees) should also receive an unknown flow of energy, by opening the small spaces behind the knees (in the popliteal coeax) that never see the light of the sun. During the day our knees are always flexed: whether walking, sitting, running or bending; therefore the backs of the knees never extend. Why not give them a chance to function again?

The back of the body is as important as the front and it must regain its dignity.

Above: The back of the lungs and ribcase, showing the deepest section of the lungs which is only penetrated by very deep inhalation.

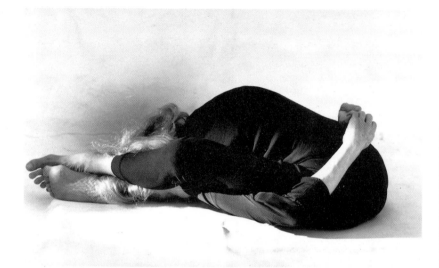

Going Round

THE IMPORTANCE OF CURVES in our daily practice.

We have to avoid angular movements and adopt circular, spiral ones. Do not attack the point you want to attain in the pose, but rather find your way to it by circling in small, light little curves (as flies and bees do when centering down, while they want to descend, aiming at a definite spot).

The body instinctively avoids all harsh and aggressive motion, dictated by pressure, leading to "fragmentary" movements; instead it accepts the rounded movements, born from the spine and therefore leading to a "total" action. This kind of "spiral-circumpheric" gesture penetrates in depth and can bring about unexpected results.

There are no beginners or advanced students – the first step is the last step. This means that fundamental principles, such as this one, are the same in all the asanas. However, they have to be clearly explained by the teacher and fully understood by the pupil.

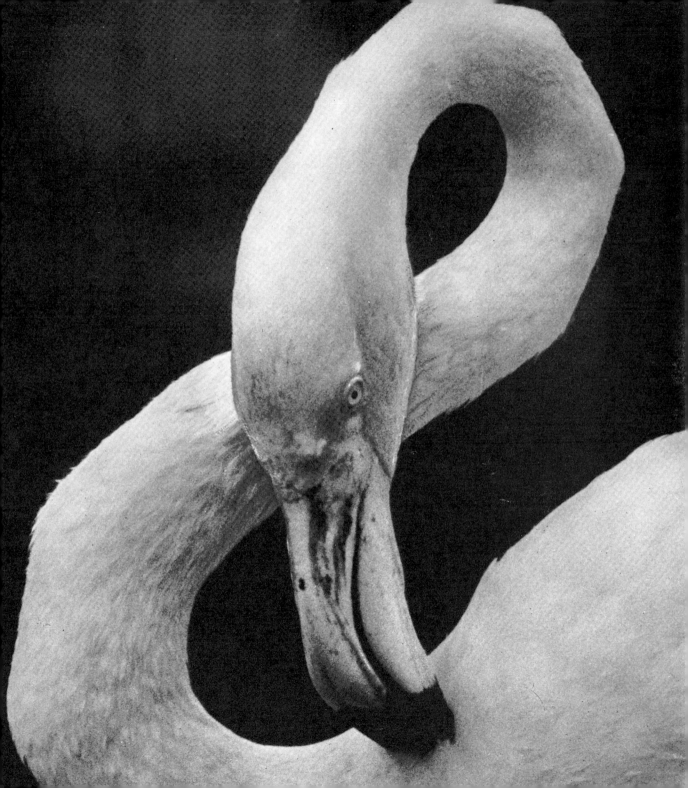

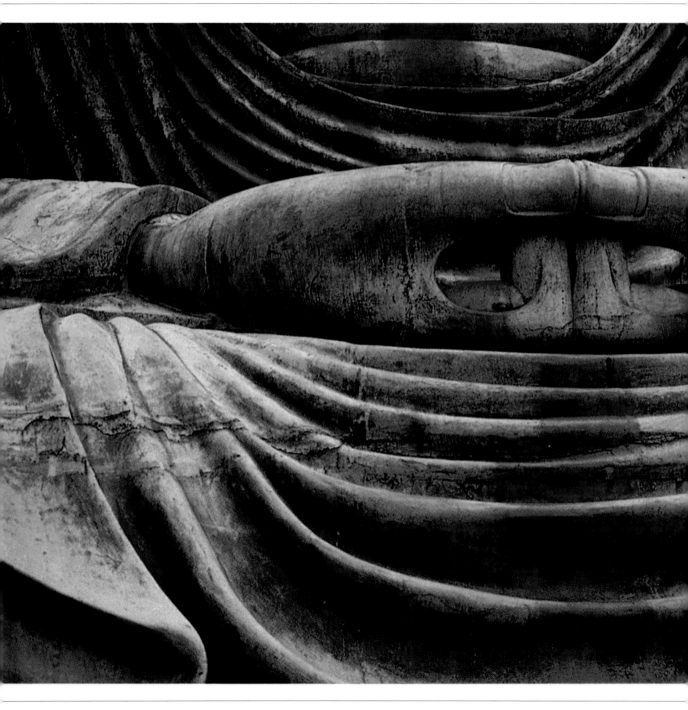

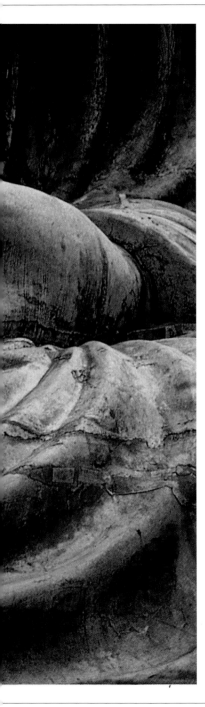

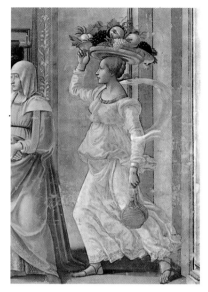

What Do We Mean By Relaxation?

TO RELAX IS NOT TO COLLAPSE, but simply to undo tension. This tension has been accumulated in the body and in the mind by years of forceful education. Tension is the result of will, effort and prejudice.

We have been trained, during the first part of our lives, to struggle to achieve. Now we have to work in the opposite direction, by letting go, giving place to a different action (if we can call it action), an "un-doing action". This will stop the habitual process of doing which has become mechanical.

The body in itself is healthy, but it has been ruined by all sorts of negative, destructive, guilt feelings. If one can avoid going in this negative direction, a positive attitude will take over and the body will then be able to start its recuperative function, its natural way of existing. There is nothing to be done. It is not a state of passivity but, on the contrary, of alert watchfulness. It is perhaps the most "active" of our attitudes, going "with" and not "against" our body and feelings.

There is beauty in the acceptance of what is.

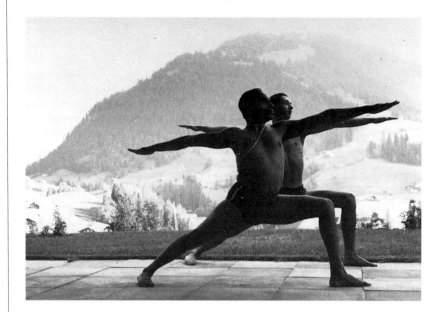

How to Practice

Above right: Vikrsāsana. *Above left:* Virabhadrāsana. The focus of yoga is the inner life of the body and āsanas should not be performed for the glory of the pose, as in classical ballet which aims solely to be a beautiful position.

I N THE BEGINNING you have to make room for yoga in your daily life, and give it the place it deserves. But after some time yoga itself will pull you up by the hair and make you do it.

Do not let your mind wander during your practice, but instead, be completely there. Let your practice be short and intense, focusing your attention on one single action, where body and brain meet at the same point at the same time.

After a lesson my students sometimes say that they are relaxed in their bodies and tired in their head. This is a good sign. With regular practice, there will be a definite improvement, bringing not only a deeper understanding, but also an increased confidence in your body.

Iyengar used to say, "*The highest point of yesterday should be the lowest point of today*".

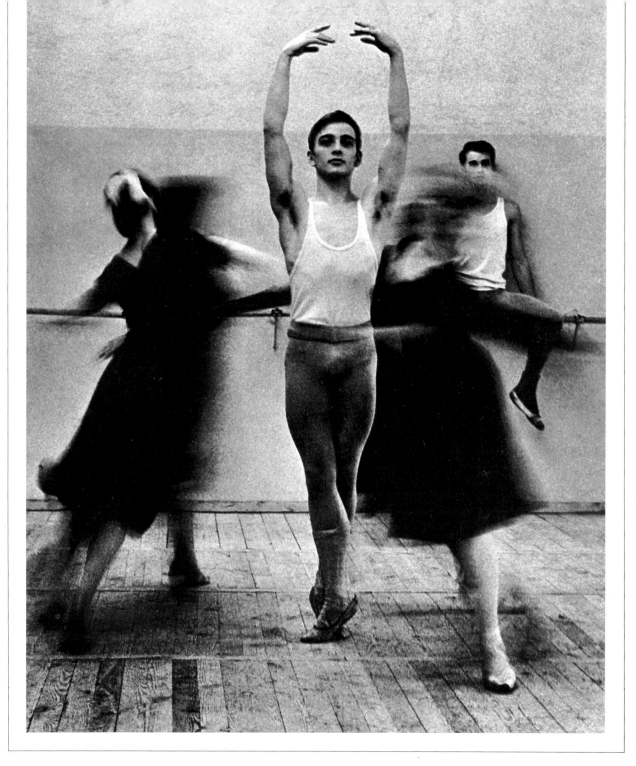

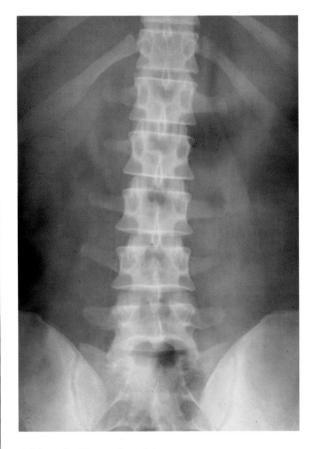

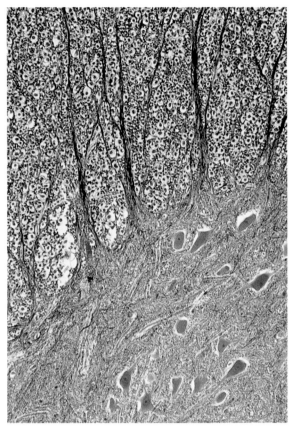

A false color X-ray of an adult lumbar and sacral vertebrae. This image includes the 12th thoracic vertebrae (on top) and below it, the five lumbar vertebrae. The spinal (which in the photograph project towards the observer) appear as elongated, oval features over the vertebral bodies.

A light micrograph of a normal human spinal cord. This cross section shows the junction between the grey matter (below, in orange) and the white matter (above).

Nerves

W HEN WE WAKE IN THE MORNING we naturally feel like stretching because the spine is beginning to extend, releasing the nerves as they become alive. The nerves get tremendous benefit from the elongation of the spine; the more extensive the lengthening, the deeper the impact and the release of the nerves.

"Everything in your body (movement, function, sensation) is controlled by your brain. Wires called nerves unite and interconnect the brain to every part of the body. These nerves carry information from the brain to the body. When you want to lift your arm, your brain sends messages along the nerves to the muscles of your arm ordering them to act." [2]

The spinal cord, protected by the vertebral column, is a very important passage and distributing station. It connects nervous energy from the central nervous system (brain) with the peripheral nervous system (nerves).

"Thirty-one pairs of spinal nerves branch from the spinal cord, with the vascular structures, and cross through the intervertebral cavities reaching the periphery.

There is not a nerve in our organism that is not, somehow, dependent on the integral functioning of the spinal cord and consequently on the vertebral column. Even the nerves of the skull, although they do not originate in the spinal cord, depend on it, since their ganglia cells receive trophic reflexes from it." [3]

This is why it is so important to focus teaching on the elongation of the spine, especially the waist area.

This lumbar area (waist vertebrae) suffers most when standing wrongly. The lumbar vertebrae that become misaligned are crushed together by tension.

These compressed vertebrae pinch the nerves that pass through the corresponding vertebral cavity, causing pain and muscular spasm.

We have to recreate the proper space between the vertebrae so that the nerves can be released and health re-established.

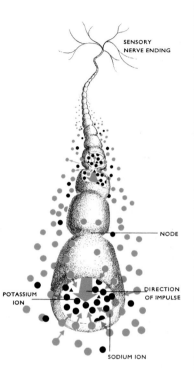

The power-house of nerves: A nerve impulse is a self-perpetuating series of electrical charges along an insulated nerve fiber. The fiber, surrounded by positive sodium ions, has potassium ions in its negative interior. Whenever a sensory nerve ending is stimulated, the sodium is temporarily admitted into the nerve as a node – a break in the insulation. The resulting electrical charge sets off a chain of charges extending from node to node to the central nervous system.

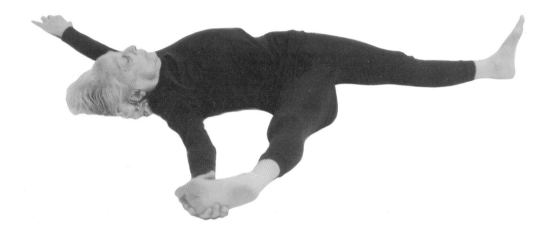

Why Are We Doing Yoga?

Above: Supta Padangusth-asāsana (one leg up, one leg down). Do not kill the instinct of the body for the glory of the pose. Do not look at your body like a stranger, but adopt a friendly approach towards it. Watch it, listen to it, observe its needs, its requests, and even have fun. To be sensitive is to be alive.

FOR HEALTH REASONS? Perhaps a walk in the park would be better. To help someone else? There are so many ways of helping people. To make money? This is surely not the best way. Out of a sense of duty and discipline? Or for some obligation towards ourselves coming from our puritanical background?

No, nothing of the kind. No motivation, no aims, only an agreeable appointment for the body to look forward to. We do it for the fun of it.

To twist, stretch, and move around, is pleasant and enjoyable, a body holiday.

There is an unexpected delight in meeting earth and sky at the same moment! (gravity).

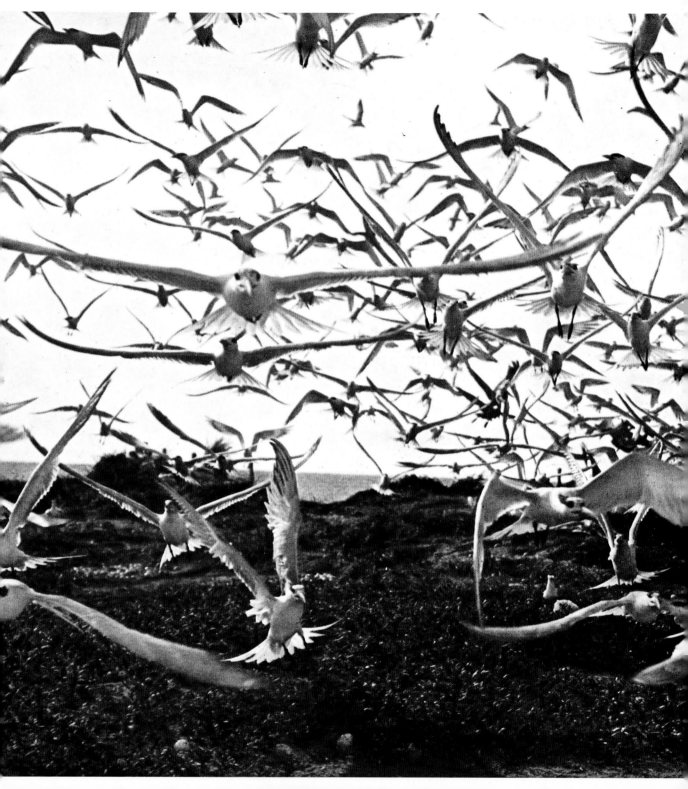

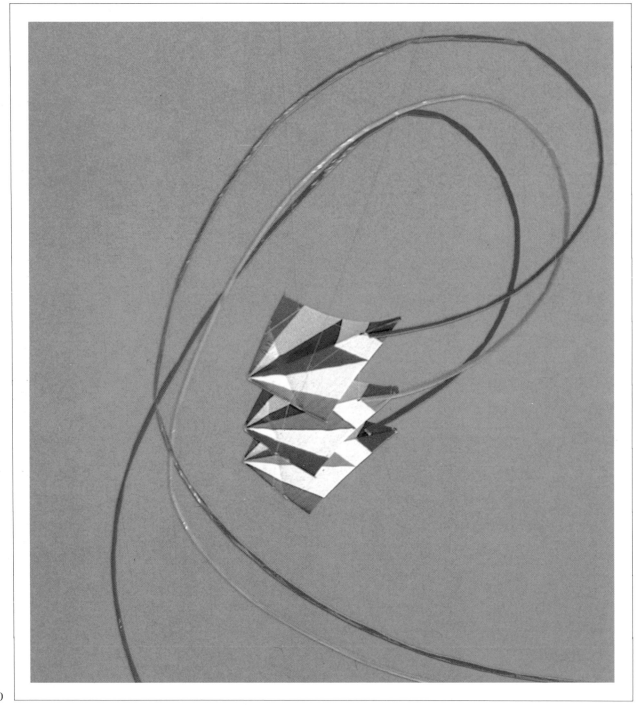

On Time

TIME IS RELATIVE. This also applies to our lives. If we are concentrated on work or on something we are interested in, it is possible that we do not realize that a couple of hours have gone by. Instead, we have the feeling only a few minutes have elapsed.

We must realize that time is a strange thing; it can dilate or shorten, in accordance with our occupations, moods, emotional state or the various images that are in our thoughts.

When we enjoy something, there is space in our brain. It is as though time became unreal and vanished. Time dilates and expands. Instead when we are in a hurry, nervous, anxious or afraid, time lessens and our frustrations seem to have no end. Also when we wait for somone we are in love with, minutes become hours. We must realize that time plays funny tricks on us like the story of Elpenor.

Elpanor was supposed to leave for Troy with Ulysses and his companions. As it was such a hot day, some hours before he had gone up to the roof of Circe's house and had fallen asleep there. When he woke up he saw that the ship was leaving so he started running after it because he did not want to be abandoned there and, forgetting that he was on a roof, dropped down from that high precipice on the void, hit his head and died. The absence of time killed him.

Einstein demonstrated how velocity influences and acts on time.

The famous Dutch physicist, Hendrik Lorentz, with his principle known as "Lorentz Contraction" explains how an object in motion and velocity diminishes, restricting its size, compressing its mass.

This phenomenon of expansion and contraction is modified by time.

Like Gods, we must have time, infinite time. Gods are not limited or restricted by time as they have a different perspective. For them, a whole life can last only a few minutes.

To have time implies that quality of elegance and ease which gives poise to our movements and wisdom to our action.

Pushed by rush, most of the time, we are compressed, mean and narrow-minded. Why not open the doors and let air, wind and sun penetrate into our hearts?

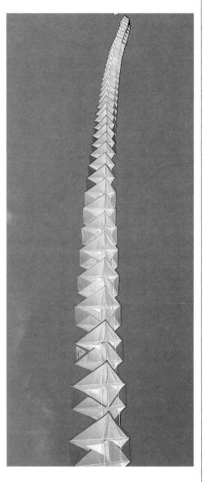

Time can dilate or shorten, depending on the attention we place upon what we are doing in any given moment. When we enjoy something, there is space in our brain and time dilates

Matter and Energy

ENERGY TRANSFORMS ITSELF into matter, as we can see every day on our planet, with its wind, water, woods, lightning, and those forms of energy derived from the sun, which have acquired a material form.

Matter transforms and changes itself into energy in which those same elements are transmuted, becoming a source of energy: wind-mills, turbines, fire, electricity, and the sun itself with its heat (being matter and energy at the same time). Sun gives life to our bodies, to animals, to trees, plants and to every living thing around us.

". . . Einstein discovered that energy is ultimately identical with matter. While those of us who are neither mathematicians nor physicists may not understand the technical implications of his theories, it is nonetheless clear that our physical bodies and our essential energy are one and the same. Our bodies are our energy: it is through the body that we move." [4]

". . . We need to consult the quantum to really understand how the mind pivots on the turning point of a molecule. A neuro-peptide springs into existence at the touch of a thought, but where does it spring from? A thought of fear and the neuro-chemical it turns into are somehow connected in a hidden process, a transformation of non-matter into matter." [5]

". . .As with the neuro-peptide, the quantum allowed nature to become flexible enough to permit the inexplicable transformation of non-matter into matter, time into space, mass into energy." [6]

Breathing and yoga exercises bring energy, transforming the body from matter into energy.

The poses (āsanas) we are doing, while breathing, give energy to our body. This energy (that comes to our body by doing the poses) gives us the possibility to act on the body.

While the process of transformation is going on, various changes are taking place in the substance of which the body is composed: in the heart, blood, lungs, bones, etc., bringing order and new vitality to the body.

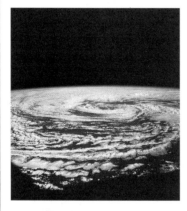

This photograph taken by Apollo 9 from space represents a storm breaking out north of Hawaii. Storms are pure energy resulting from the interaction of different atmospheric bodies and manifest themselves in matter; heavy rain, strong winds, lightning and thunder. *Opposite*: This meteor crater in Arizona is perhaps the earth's most studied impact structure. Nearly a mile across and originally 750 feet deep, the crater – here encrusted by snow – is attributed to a 300,000-ton meteorite some 50,000 years ago. Meteorites of this size, which can unleash the explosive energy of nuclear weapons, probably fall less than once every thousand years.

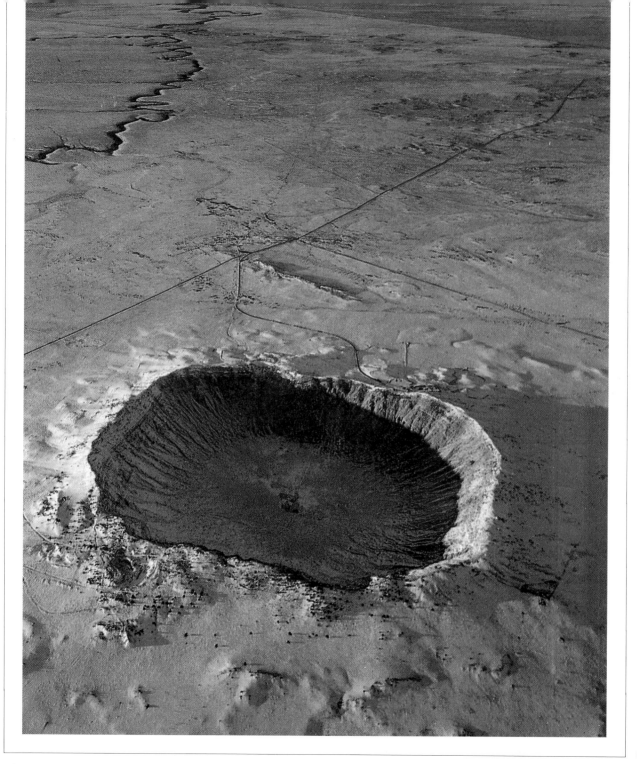

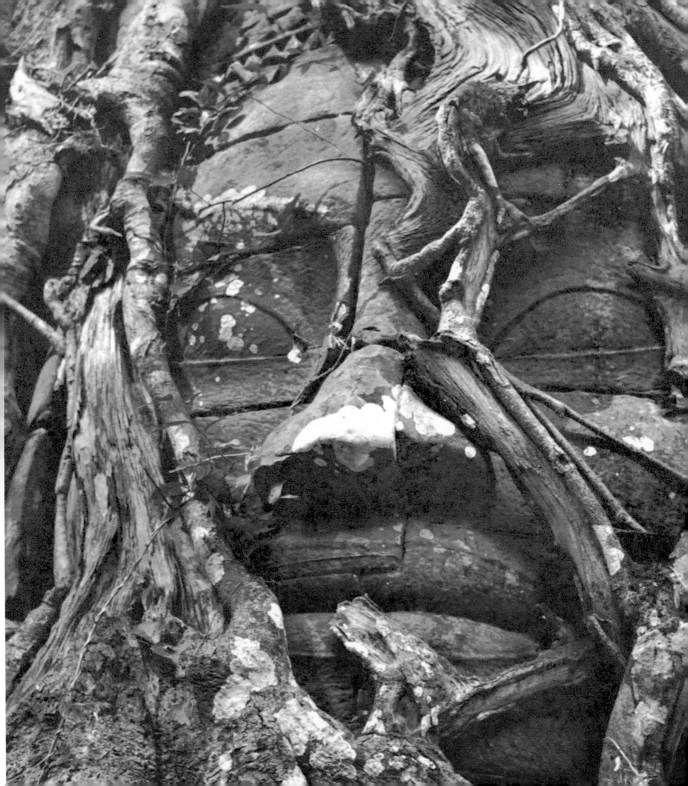

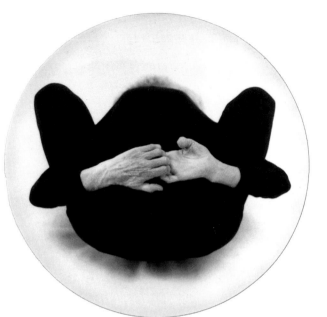

The Importance of Daily Practice

Above: Supta Kurmāsana (Tortoise). *Opposite:* The gods are not merciful about our distractions or our absent-mindedness. The image of a godhead overgrown by plants in a tropical forest.

AFTER THE FIRST BURST of enthusiasm, often we slack our practice, forgetting the many advantages already obtained through the improvement of our health.

Instead, in this kind of work, continuity and perseverance are required. We will progress much more effectively through daily training. When we are not well we turn to our practice. But perhaps, illness could have been prevented, avoided or even totally rejected, if we had kept our body in full health by practicing.

The gods are not merciful about our distractions or our absent-mindedness. When we have seen light in a certain direction, we have to go further with it and follow the grain until the end of the journey.

When truth has been revealed to us, we cannot go back into the old pattern with our usual silly mistakes. No excuses can be accepted, no justifications can be offered, life is too demanding and we have to hold it in our hands.

In reference to this, there is a good old Indian story that Krishnamurti loved to tell.

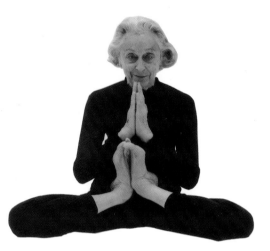

Above: Kandasana. *Opposite*: Meditation and awareness can be found even in the ordinary act of walking. To make a decision and to follow it through to the the very end requires single-minded focus and clarity.

It is about a young man and Vishnu.

A disciple, feeling very thankful and wanting to please his teacher, asked what he could do to demonstrate his gratitude and devotion.

The day was very hot and Vishnu answered: "*Will you please bring me a glass of water?*"

Very surprised about that simple request, the disciple left and went to the well to fill a glass with water.

There he saw, sitting on the edge of the well, a lovely young woman and, falling in love with her, he forgot everything else.

Time passed and with time his life. He had a lot of adventures, traveled, married, had children and so on.

Many years later, during the season of rains, finding himself in a tremendous flood, with his family around on the point of drowning, while his grand-children were screaming clasping his hairs on the top of his head, he desperately invoked Vishnu for help.

Vishnu, peeping from the thunder clouds answered him:

"*Where is my glass of water?*"

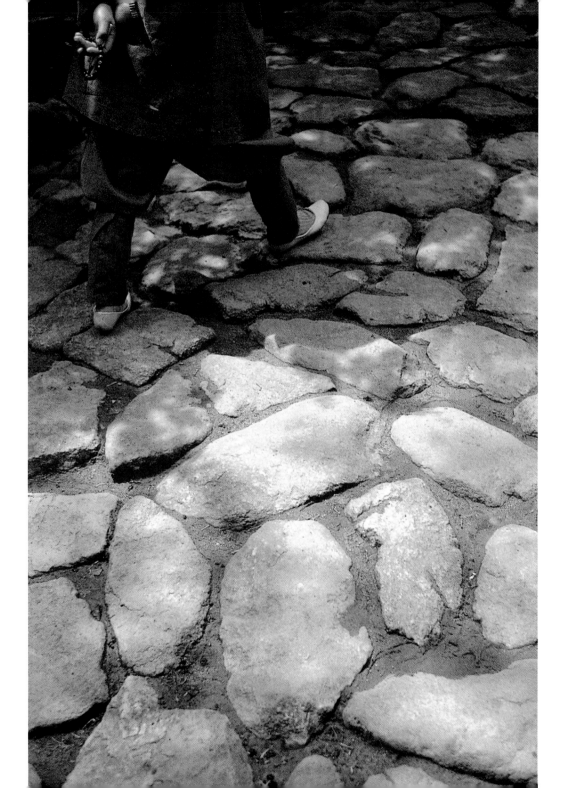

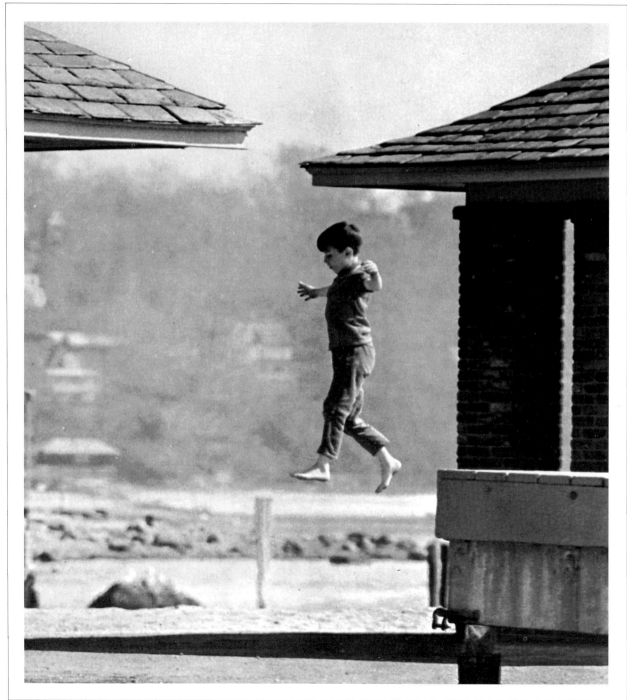

The Heel in Greek Mythology

THERE ARE MANY STORIES about this part of the foot in Greek history. The heel is a very particular and special spot in our body. In ancient times, especially in Greek mythology, this part of the body had an important place in their tradition.

Achilles, the Greek hero familiar to us all, Oedipus, Philoctetes, and even Zeus (the tendons of whose feet were cut by Typhon,[7] as Paul Diel mentions) all were damaged in their heels.

Paul Diel says "*The foot represents the state and destiny of the soul*" [8] and an infirmity in this very spot can be interpreted as a disconnection between man and the universe.

When the body is unbalanced it leads to all sorts of unhappiness and misery.

Oedipus

Oedipus' history and myth is the result of a psychological muddle, an involution of normality, killing his father and marrying his mother!!

He had a good brain, but the brain cannot function by itself without that magic flow, it works uselessly and moves in a void. That flow of life (from the heels to the top of the head) which brings energy and order in our brain, in us, and consequently around us, is essential. This "connection" is of the greatest importance: it is the connection of earth to sky, of matter to brain, the link from human to the divine and also from heaviness to lightness in our body. It is all produced by gravity, which corresponds in the trees and plants to the movement from the roots towards the sun.

Oedipus' distortion can perhaps be restored by order. To transcend this disorder, one needs the mysterious divine touch which can readjust and transmute the cause. Therefore our life should be inspired and our actions, as well as the motives behind them, should be dedicated to others.

Only this "*otherness*" can correct us and save us from an unhappy destiny. [9]

Opposite: A small boy jumps from a beach float. The foot is a very strong ensemble of bones and muscles which supports the whole body even against the shock of a landing after jumping.

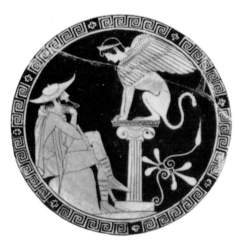

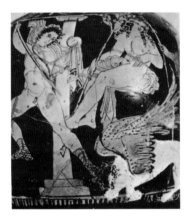

Above center: Oedipus as a
bearded traveller contemplates
a sculpture of the Sphinx.
Above: Oedipus slaying the
Sphinx watched over by
Apollo.

As Saint Paul says : "*We must make this corruptible body incorruptible*". [10]

"*. . . Oedipus' father Laios, having been warned by the oracle, fears that his son Oedipus will oust him and kill him upon reaching adulthood. The child is exposed to the mountains so that he may perish.*"

"*. . . Laios has the tendons of the infant's feet cut before exposing him.*"

"*. . . In contrast to Zeus, Oedipus remains crippled. His soul can be cured only with the help of the spirit-Zeus: help which is granted him only according to the extent of his own spiritual endeavors (efforts towards a higher consciousness).*

The wounded foot is of primary importance in the story and it is emphasized by the very name of the hero: Oedipus means "he who limps" (the literal translation is "swollen foot", which indicates a soul swollen with vanity). Oedipus will not pass through life with a sprintly gait." [11]

Philoctetes

This hero has been a puzzle for many historians because there are different interpretations of his legend. Philoctetes, son of Peante, (from poia, poa, "grass", shepherd) King of Melida, walking on mount Eta in Thessaly, was looking for his flock and found Heracles on the pyre that had been built for him. He was in agony because none of his

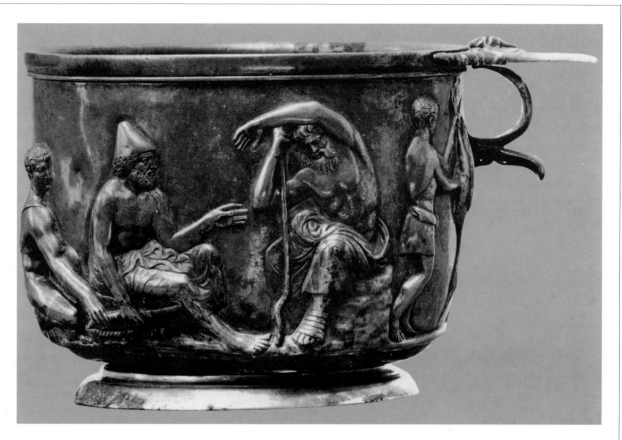

followers wanted to ignite the fire while he was still alive. Heracles gave Philoctetes his bow and poisoned arrows in exchange for agreeing to light the fire.

Philoctetes was one of Helen's suitors. He brought seven ships to the war of Troy and was at the head of the expedition.

When they arrived in Tenedo, they decided to make a sacrifice to Apollo on the island of Crise, to gain Apollo's mercy and while they were in the temple, a snake from the sea bit Philoctetes' foot. The pain was terrible, the wound became infected and the bad smell disturbed the crew. Philoctetes complained so much they became sick of him, and under Ulysses' advice, they left him on the island of Lemno, while the ships went back to Troy under Medonate's guidance.

Odysseus is shown on this silver cup trying to convince Philocetes to return to Troy. The dejected hero is shown with a bandaged foot and staff.

71

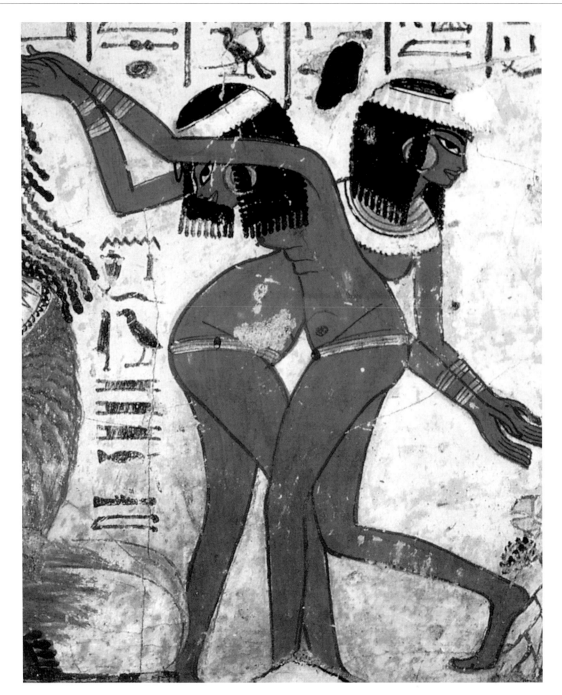

Thanks to the bow and arrows he received from Heracles, he survived by hunting birds and wild animals that he could find.

Ten years later, Ulysses, at the suggestion of the fortune teller Eleno (who told him that Troy would never be taken until Philoctetes came back with Heracle's bow) decided to act with Neoptolemus, Achilles' son, went to persuade Philoctetes to come back to Troy to fight the Trojans.

Neoptolemus was also angry with the Greeks because they had refused to give him his father's (Achilles) shield. So a liaison developed between Philoctetes and Neoptolemus. And Neoptolemus agreed to take Philoctetes home to Athens.

At that point Heracles also came into the story and told Philoctetes he must return to Troy because of his duty to the community. Philoctetes left the island. But before reaching Troy they stopped at Aesculeppius, the island where the god of healing was born, to cure Philoctetes' foot.

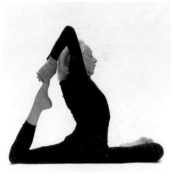

Later on, while in Troy, Philoctetes killed Paris with one of his poisoned arrows.*

The legend says that the serpent was the guardian of the temple and bit Philoctetes in order to protect that sacred place, which should not have been profaned by strangers.

Some maintain that the envy of his companions hung over him like a persecution, because he possessed the bow and arrows of Eracle.

Above: Ekapada Rajakapotāsana.

Left: Egyptian Celebrants.

Or perhaps the Gods, on the Olympus, claiming him or his father responsible for Eracle's death, required that he should suffer and be punished for all those years of purification with a wound on one of the most vital parts of the body. The heroes of the Gods are not permitted transgressions.

Remember that the "art of Yoga" (as Iyengar calls it) implies a severe austerity: and, at the same time, a joyfulness, in each day of life. There is an Italian expression "Allegrezza" (which we find also in the Bible). Saint Paul says, "...*E qualunque cosa facciate, fatela con animo*", "...*And whatever thing you do, do it with good will (happiness, in a happy mood)*" (12)

* This second part of the story is taken from Sophocles version of the tragedy. One can give all manner of psychological and symbolic interpretations to this strange story that feed the imagination, but the problem of Philoctetes, abandoned in that Island with his wounded heel, remains unsolved.

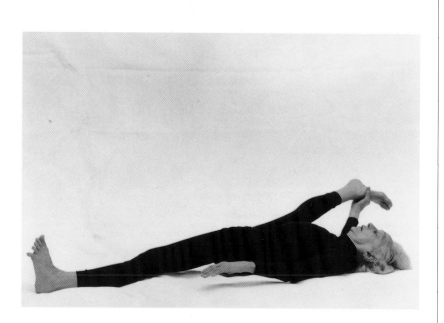

Achilles

Thetis, Goddess of the Sea, after Achilles' birth, lifted him by one leg, keeping his heel in her hand and dipped him into the sea, so that he would become strong, healthy and invulnerable. Only one part of his body remained out of water: the heel that she was holding between her fingers. At that very point he remained vulnerable. If an arrow would hit there he would die. And so it happened.

(Witness also Achilles' vulnerable foot, which symbolizes the vulnerability of his soul, his inclination towards anger, the cause of his downfall). [13]

The heel, and in particular the very back of the heel (where Thetis' fingers hold Achilles' foot), is a vulnerable spot. It is a vital delicate part that sustains and holds us, and on which (in line with the spine) we are able to rely.

If one uses it in the right way, in tune with gravity, somehow it will protect the body, making it, if not invulnerable, at least less vulnerable.

The heel is a very vulnerable spot as the legend of Achilles and Teti testifies. By using the heel in the right way with the force of gravity, it will become stronger and thus be able to protect the body. *Above:* Supta Trivikāsana. The heel grounds the whole body and maintains the constant contact with the earth. *Opposite:* The roots of a tree on autumn ground. The heel could be compared to the roots of the tree for it is essential in the contact with the force of gravity that pulls us towards the ground.

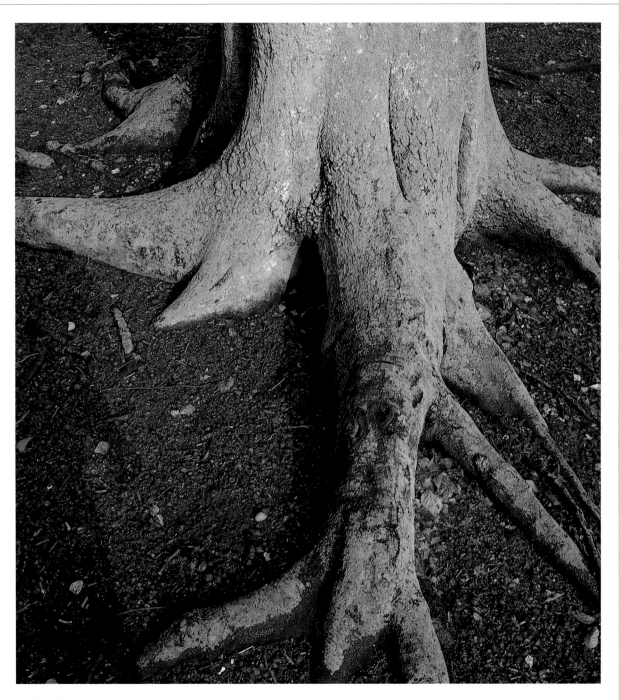

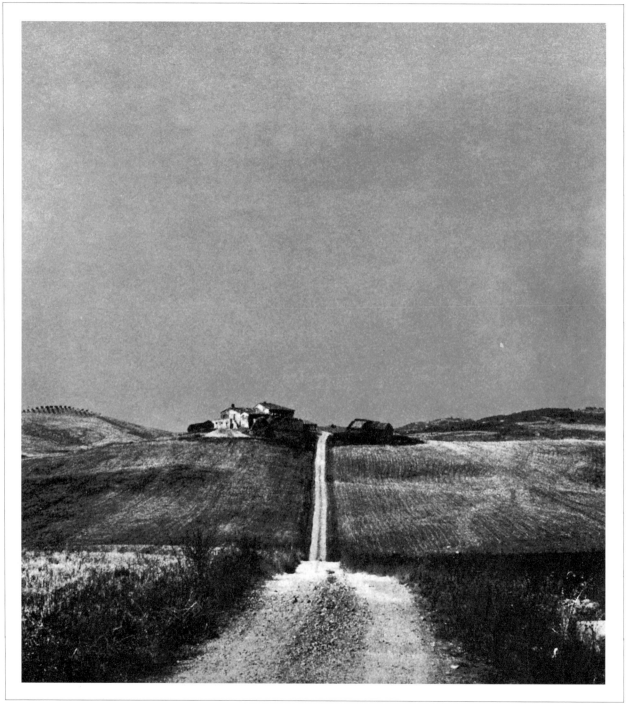

On Memory and Age

MEMORY IS CONNECTED WITH ATTENTION. An attentive mind remembers. A distracted mind forgets. Attention is energy and produces energy when we use it. It is like the battery in a car, that recharges itself in the running of the motor.

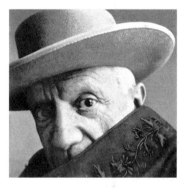

There is no physical or intellectual energy, there is only energy. It is not a question of age, being young or old, it is a question of intensity.

Goethe wrote the "*Faust*" when he was already in advanced age. Richard Wagner composed his "*Parsifal*" at 80 years of age and the sparkling opera of Giuseppe Verdi, "*Falstaff*", was written by him after he was 80.

Many "*Requiems*" composed by musicians at the end of their lives were considered among their best works.

Toscanini at 80 years old led his orchestra with such intensity and vigor that other young conductors would watch with astonishment.

And what about Victor Hugo who died at 83 and started to write "*Les Miserables*" at 60?

Picasso's vivacity after he was 90 was proverbial.

The best talks given by Jiddu Krishnamurti were delivered after his seventies. He was like fire when he wanted to convey something he cared for and the public were often shaken by his words. The urge to communicate was so strong in him that even the atmosphere in the room changed when he was talking.

Opposite: the ageless appeal of an old farm in Tuscany. *Above:* A portrait of Picasso; his genius seemed to increase with his age.

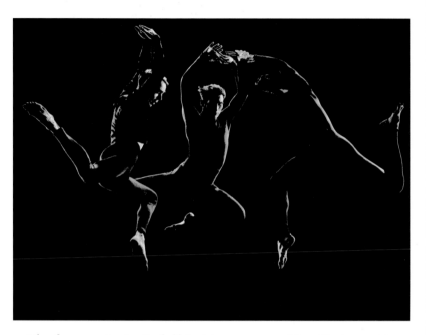

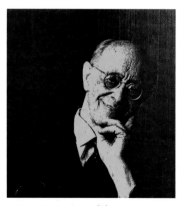

Above: A portrait of the pianist Rudolf Serkin. *Top of this page*: "*Centaurus*", a picture framing pure energy in action.

Opposite: Arturo Toscanini, the conductor.

The famous pianist Rudolf Serkin, now over 90, still plays with an astonishing fervor and the strength he is able to convey through the rigorousness of his rhythm is quite amazing.

We all have in mind the divine voice of Pablo Casals' cello. He was over 90 but his enthusiasm, freshness, purity and naivete never left him. He remained young until the end of his life. He had the possibility to bring us with him to the mysterious world where miracles still happen and each of his concerts was a miracle, for the simplicity, depth and beauty that he expressed through the music he was playing.

All these formidable brains were working at high speed until the end of their life.

Here are only a few samples among the great many that could be given. Those people continue to live intensely even at an old age. With their power of concentration and the passion for their art (burning as fire in them) they are capable of modifying the physical limitations by which the body is conditioned. The efficiency of an attentive mind is incalculable.

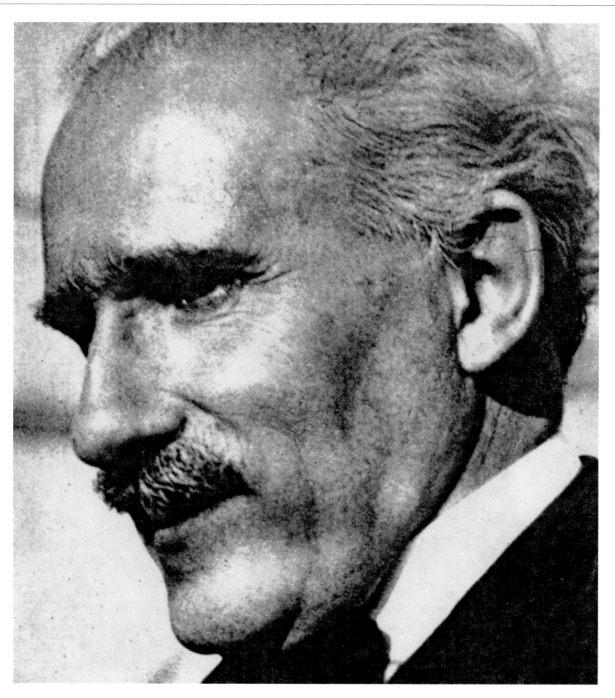

The old seem often to forget, but it is only that they are not interested in what they are doing. They lose contact with the world, with their environment, with themselves. They too easily give up their activities and the things they care for, taking refuge in their own protective shell.

We have to keep on using and entertaining our memory. It is a delicate organ and must be looked after with care.

Do not press your brain to remember, on the contrary, give it time, relax it.

Why do we want to remember? If we forget we forget, we are going to remember when we least expect it. Can we not see that it is the fear not to remember that paralyzes the brain?

The full blossoming of maturity is the best fruit that life can offer. The need to become is over. Can we not feel the beauty to be what we are in total acceptance?

The body has its own memory and after the yoga poses (through which you are not pushed but invited to collaborate) and especially during the night, it continues to work in its joyful expansion.

The delight of the body's unfolding is surprising. Even the pores of the skin, in their slow opening, seem to participate with the rest of the body.

We forget things collected mechanically by the brain but we easily remember events in which we are somehow emotionally wrapped. They remain, painted with vivid colors.

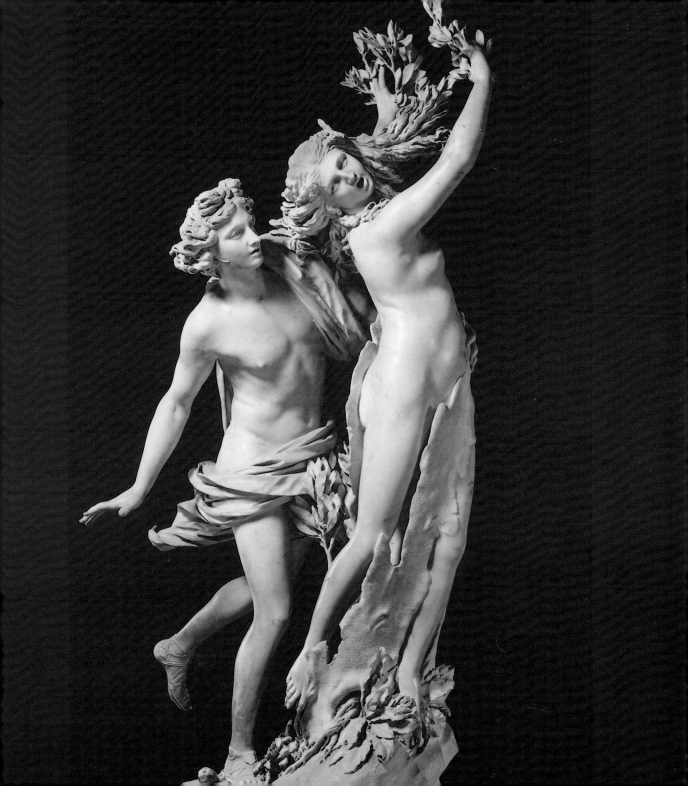

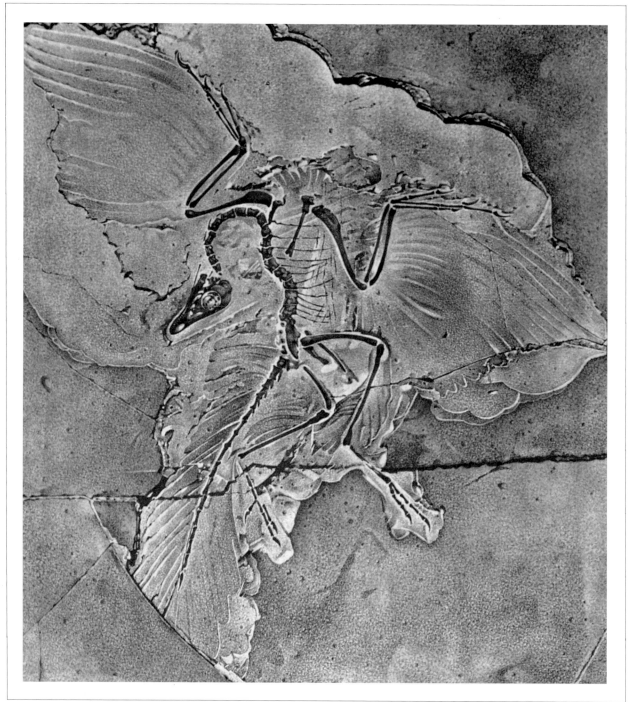

The psychological impact of a memory is more important than the fact itself, because where the sensations are involved there is a deeper and stronger connection. This will affect the unconscious, leaving a mark in the memory which may pop up spontaneously, like a spring, when required.

Marcel Proust described a "madeleine" (the little French cake) in the beginning of his book – "*A La Recherche Du Temps Perdu*" – where the taste of it during the breakfast of Monsieur Swann, awakens in his memory many sensations, bringing him back to his childhood.

People remember salient moments of their life; exciting moments where beauty and love were condensed. But they also like to sink back, reminiscing and talking about unpleasant events: the war, the death of someone they cherished, their illness and so on, where they have been psychologically hurt and where fear was present.

They hold those wounds like precious jewels. It is a weight that does not drop easily from their shoulders.

The part of the brain in which memory resides is paved with all sorts of images, most of the past, covering it like a veil. When something new is dropped in that thick layer of thoughts and sensations, it is obviously more difficult to remember. Such an occupied container is not free to receive, as all sorts of distractions are interfering. Instead, when there is space one retains and remembers more easily.

Why does memory absorb like a sponge? Why do we retain? Perhaps because our lives are sometimes so empty, insignificant and shallow and memory grasps hold of the few things we lived intensely, sticking to them.

Memory is there. It contains our past conditioning: our childhood, our education, our culture (from which our taste is molded), our experiences, our knowledge, our environment, our country, our family, our friends. Let us leave all this alone and not use those things, not exploit them or speculate upon them. They should remain there in complete immobility like the background of a picture or a map.

Opposite: A clay print of the "Archaeopteryxthe", the earliest known bird whose features were almost reptilian. Old memories remain imprinted in our brain for years, almost like fossils, for the psychological impact of a memory is more important than the fact itself.

Below: Fragments of a "Khata" a ritual shawl, entangled with spring blossom at Tashilhumpo monastery in Tibet. *Opposite:* Prayer flags stand in the Kyichu River near Lhasa, capital of Tibet.

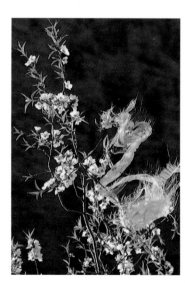

Not to carry them along is a blessing! With the purpose of pointing out the beauty of a fresh mind, Krishnamurti told this story :

The story concerns two monks traveling by foot together. On their way they meet a woman sitting beside a river. She asks them to help her to cross the stream. Courteously, they lift her up, putting her on their shoulders and, with the water up to their knees, after reaching the other side of the river, they lay her gently down. Then they keep on walking silently along the road. After some time, one of the monks asks his friend: "Was it not a sin to take her in our arms?" The other monk answers "You still carry her on? I left her a long time ago!"

Meeting of Body and Mind

WE MUST REALIZE that it is no longer time for us to be concerned with military training. Such things have been important from the beginning of times until this century. Now this form of conscription is no longer really felt. Young people do not want it any more, it does not interest them. The urge to defend the country against the enemy is gone. Instead we feel a desire for universality and community born into the new generations. They are against wars, against conflicts.

With airplanes one can, in a few hours, circle around the world. Space and distance no longer separate countries and people meet without the old prejudices of races and colors.

Sports are now taking over, but this intolerable fever where ambition and exhibitionism have the most important place, where athletes are ruled and pulled by competition, where the body becomes an instrument for an achievement (strife) to reach a certain standard or goal (so that they can improve their career in order to obtain prestige and success, not to mention money) is not dignified. It is a physical mortification.

In the meantime young people are victims of a forceful, brutal violence and often damage themselves as a result.

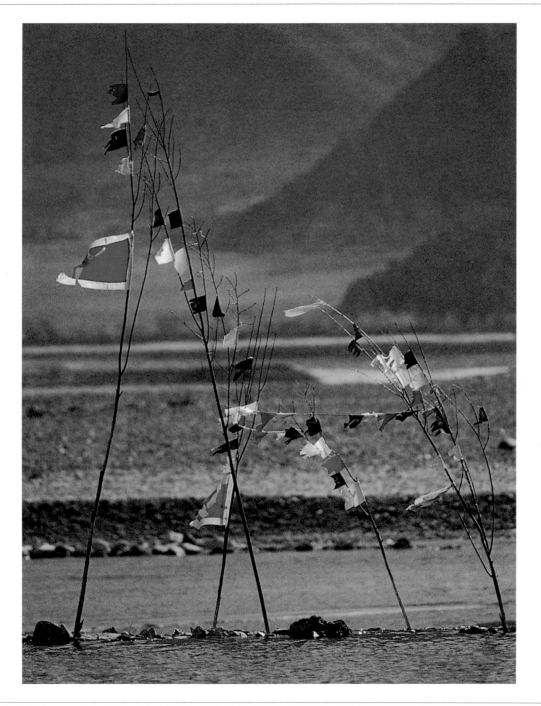

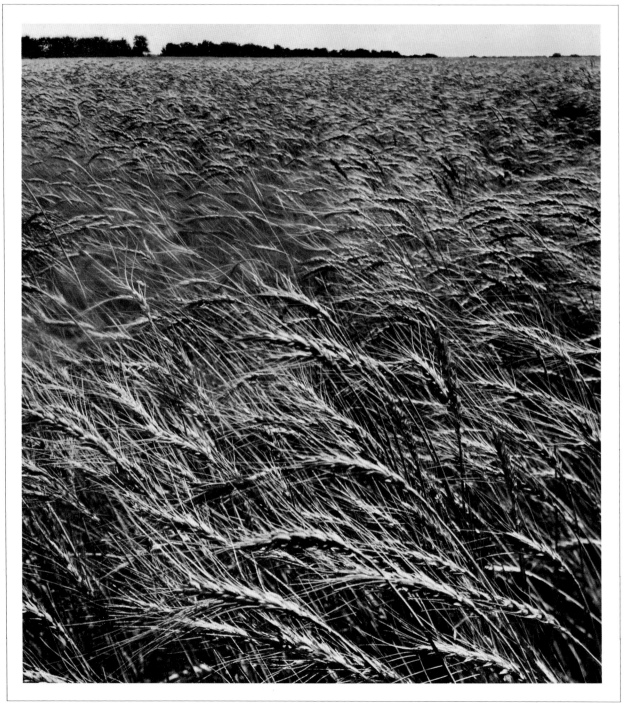

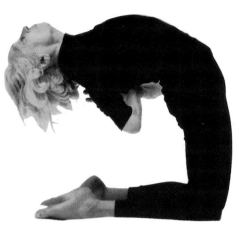

Above: Ekapada Rajakapotāsana.

We work *against* the body, not *with* the body. When we work with the body there is beauty, there is harmony. As the Greek philosopher Alcmaeon, of the school of Croton, maintained: "Health is harmony; disease is a disturbance of harmony." *

"*. . . The mind and the body are so intimately connected that ultimately we cannot tell the difference between them. Ultimately, indeed, they tell the same stories about us. But the body is the more visible aspect of the being and so may speak for itself. When we align the body we also align the mind. The body is the hologram of the being, as Alexander Lowen has said. 'The body does not lie'*" [14]

The body needs the mind and the mind needs the body. The body must remain pure, untouched, not "used". Why do we hurt ourselves? Why do we sacrifice the body for the sake of ideas, for the "ultimate cause"? Even if it is the ultimate, it is always a cause.

No self-centered attitude, no self-immolation, no violence against ourselves, all these things belong to the past and it is an old-fashioned way of behaving. Why not be like the flowers in the field without any reason? They live, they blossom, they expand. Their perfume is swept in the air by the wind and it is not contaminated by ideas, duties, motivations. Those things would twist the flowers in different directions.

* A younger member of the Croton school (possibly of the fifth century A.D.) was Alcmaeon, whose principal focus was on man, not on the cosmos. His work "Concerning Nature" may be the beginning of Greek medical literature, but only a few fragments survive. Works by a number of later writers – especially Aristotle – are the principal sources for what was contained in Alcmaeon's teachings. ". . . His combination of direct observation and experimental testing stands out as unique in his time." [15]

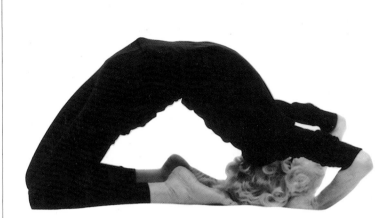

Why is it that we cannot simply exist? Why can we not do things for the sake of doing them? As Kant said, *"....Fur das ding in sich"* (....for the thing in itself).

Even the worship of gurus, teachers, priests is over. Denial is the result of a good mind that is not afraid to explore.

Is it possible to have a different attitude in which a new intelligence, not imposed by authority, but born from interest, attention and sensitivity, will emerge and in which body and mind, fused in one single action, are collaborating together?

It is just this revolutionary attitude that we are going to discover through a new discipline in the practice of yoga.

Opposite: Ostrakon with colored drawing of an Egyptian dancer. circa 1180 BC.

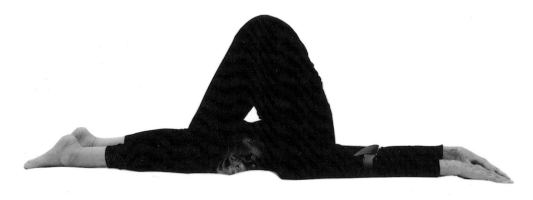

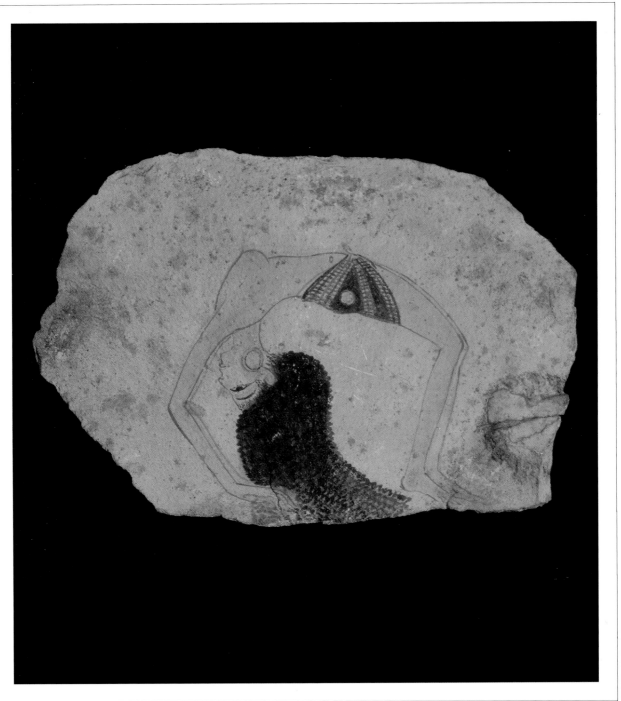

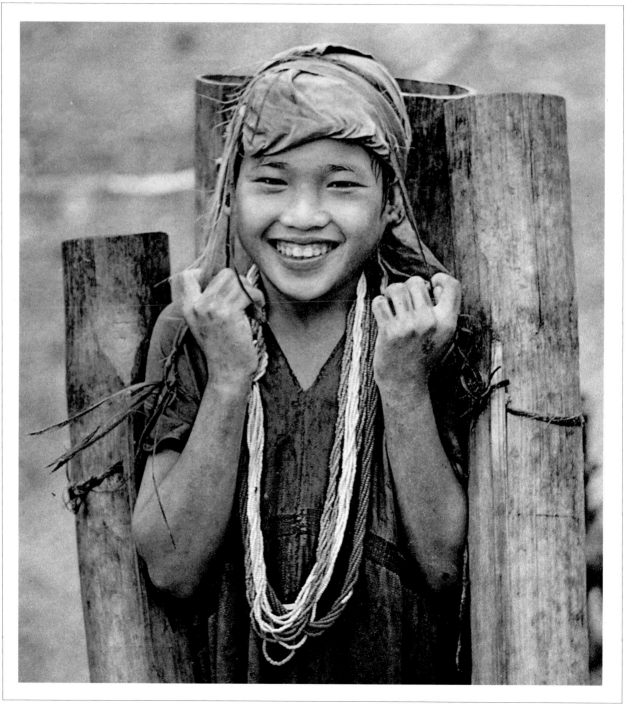

On Beauty

THERE IS NO BEAUTY WITHOUT LOVE and there is no love without beauty.

What is beauty? Are love and beauty interconnected? Does beauty derive from love? Or does love derive from beauty?

You will discover the amazing transformation in a person when she is loved, she blossoms, becoming more beautiful each day.

When we love what we are doing there is beauty in it and even the more insignificant work becomes attractive.

Love has no barriers, it is like a pool spring, pouring water endlessly. And it is perhaps this absence of limitation that gives wings to fly.

Beauty is the absence of a definite determined action, the freedom from slavery to an already formed ideal that drives us in a particular direction eliminates all other possibilities to wander among the many adventurous, and sometimes dangerous, roads. Beauty gives also the pleasure to uncover and the luxury to lose.

Is beauty mysteriously hidden behind the feeling of the unknown? To discover, to find out, to leave behind is fascinating. Is there anything more attractive in life than making the impossible possible?

"... When someone is seeking" said Siddhartha, "it happens quite easily that he only sees the thing that he is seeking; that he is unable to find anything, unable to absorb anything because he is only thinking of the thing he is seeking, because he has a goal, because he is obsessed with his goal. Seeking means: to have a goal; but finding means: to be free, to be receptive, to have no goal. You, O worthy one, are perhaps indeed a seeker, for in striving towards your goal, you do not see many things that are under your nose." [16]

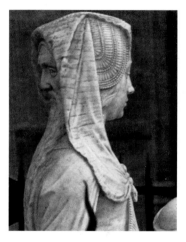

Above: Youth and Beauty, Age and Wisdom are twin aspects in this Janus like head from Spain. *Opposite*: A young Thai tribes-girl carrying bamboo.

91

Beauty is relative. Our sense of beauty is conditioned by our taste. We can react to the taste of the environment by which we have been influenced during our childhood, or we can accept it and lean on it.

We in the West may simply enjoy a vase of flowers whereas for the Japanese it can appear phony for they have a special tradition and art to flower arranging. Their gardens are so different from ours. They respond to a particular architecture the charm of which we miss. The same principle applies to a picture that may be lovely for one person and ugly for another, simply because of a different development.

Western buildings of the fourteen hundreds or Michelangelo's paintings and sculptures cannot be understood deeply and fully by everybody. Each one is looking through his own background, therefore beauty does not respond to a definite, absolute model. It is the result of our conditioning.

In some sports only a part of the body is developed, for example the arm in tennis, the legs in football, the twist of the hips in golf, where one single side of the body is extended along the leg and arm. This will unbalance the structure of our bones and create a disharmony in our movements.

A musician will adjust his arms, hands and fingers in accordance with the instrument he is playing, making only one part of the body alive and sensitive. But in yoga the physical adjustment to the poses is total, we play with our whole body. There is unity in the different members where all of them participate working together in the same time. This is the beauty of it.

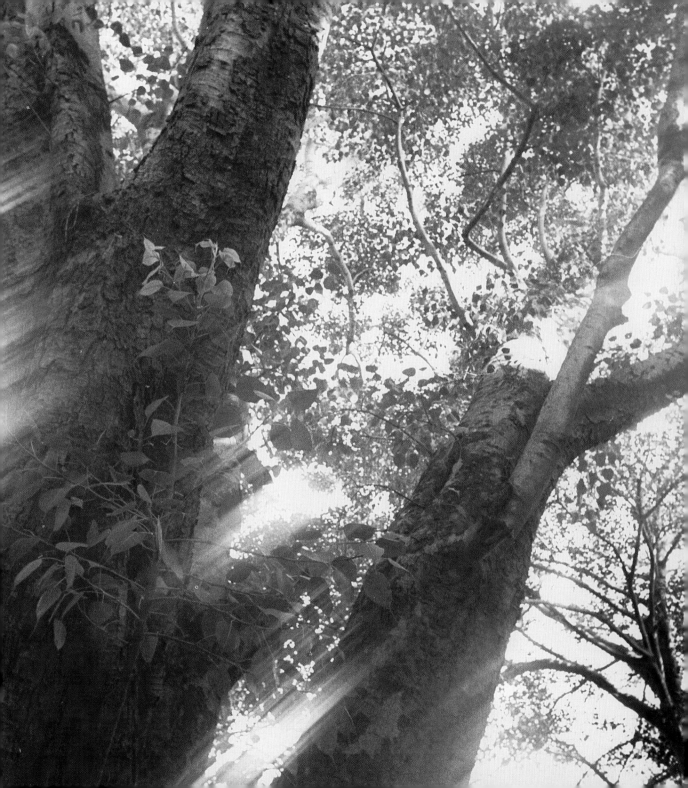

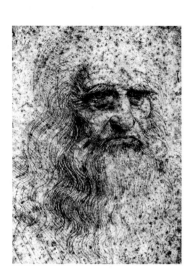

It is evident that a child will learn a piece of music more quickly where there is melody, rather than an exercise in which only technique is required. Therefore beauty comes first.

In the same way, yoga will be accepted by the body when it is done without resistance. The wave along the spine is like the melody in music. When the beautiful flow of extension is in action, this wave (felt along the magical attraction of gravity) will help the body find the right adjustment in the performance of the various movements.

There is also great beauty in following, while breathing, the slow spreading of the lungs so delicate and, at the same time, so powerful, bringing life into all of us.

Leonardo da Vinci thought that in the future he would be remembered for his inventions: the many machines he created, the aqueduct he built when he was in Milan, the researches he did in the anatomic field by studying and drawing so precisely the many different parts of the human body, the attempts to fly, and so on. But instead, he owes most of his glory to the very few pictures he painted and he remained famous because of the great "beauty" condensed in them.

Left: the famous portrait of Leonardo de Vinci. *Opposite:* One of the most striking portrayals of beauty. The great master owes most of his glory to the very few pictures he painted for the great beauty that is condensed in them.

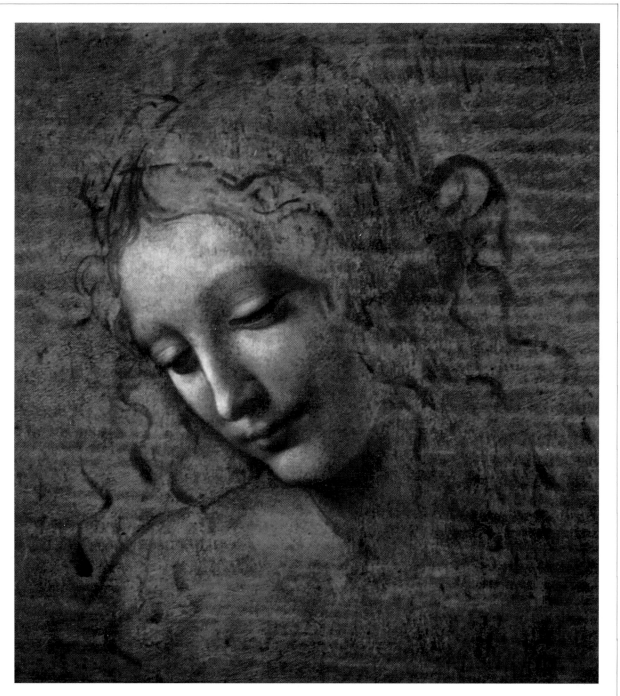

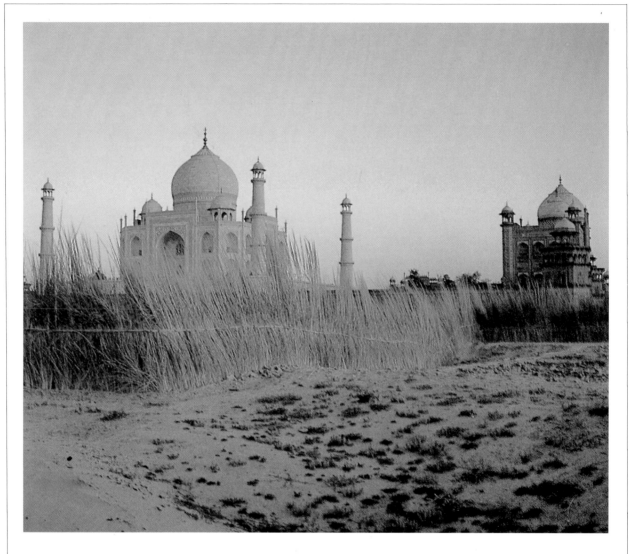

Above: The Taj Mahal, India.
Throughout the ages temples
have been erected and religious
poetry written simply as
expressions of inner and outer
beauty.

Beauty is not only in the spectacular glow of a sunset, in the delightful face of a child, in the incredible structure of a flower, in the joy of bright colors, in the shape of a sculpture, in the words of a poem, in the voice of a song, in the notes of a symphony. There is beauty also in the acknowledgment and expression of a feeling, in the logical process of thinking, in the discovery of a truth, in the realization of harmony, in the astonishment arising from observing the perfection with which a tree or a plant is put together. In the absence of fear (not in courage, courage being the opposite of fear, therefore a reaction), in the absence of noise (outside and inside us), in the violence of the wind, or in the fury of a storm.

Beauty brings us back that state of vulnerability, innocence and abandon in which, like a child, we are taken by the hand to disclose the kingdom of wonders and marvels thus putting us in touch with Nature where the miracle of existence is renewed each day.

We need beauty around us. Beauty is like a perfume impalpable but yet so very strong. Beauty is the essence of life. Its feeling pushes the artist to create, opens the heart to love, leads the brain to clarify, invites the mind to comprehend and brings the body to participate.

You find yourself in Beauty, unexpectedly absorbed by Beauty.

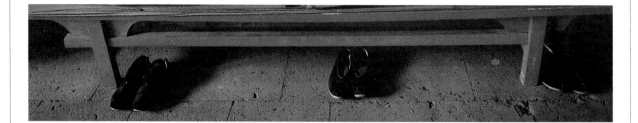

The Foot in the Chinese Tradition

"The true man breathes with his heels."

Above: The shoes of Chinese Buddhist monks are carefully put away under a bench. *Opposite:* A mural ideogram of Tibetan Buddhism.

EXCERPT FROM *Chuang Tzu*, Chapter 6, "The Great Venerable Teacher":

What do I mean by a true man? The True Man of ancient times did not rebel against want, did not grow proud in plenty, and did not plan his affairs. A man like this could commit an error and not regret it, could meet with success and not make a show. A man like this could climb high places and not be frightened, could enter the water and not get wet, could enter the fire and not get burned. His knowledge was able to climb all the way up to the Way like this.

The True Man of ancient times slept without dreaming and woke without care; he ate without savoring and his breath came from deep inside. The True Man breathes with his heels; the mass of men breathe with their throats. Crushed and bound down, they gasp their words as though they were retching. Deep in their passions and their desires, they are shallow in the workings of Heaven." [17]

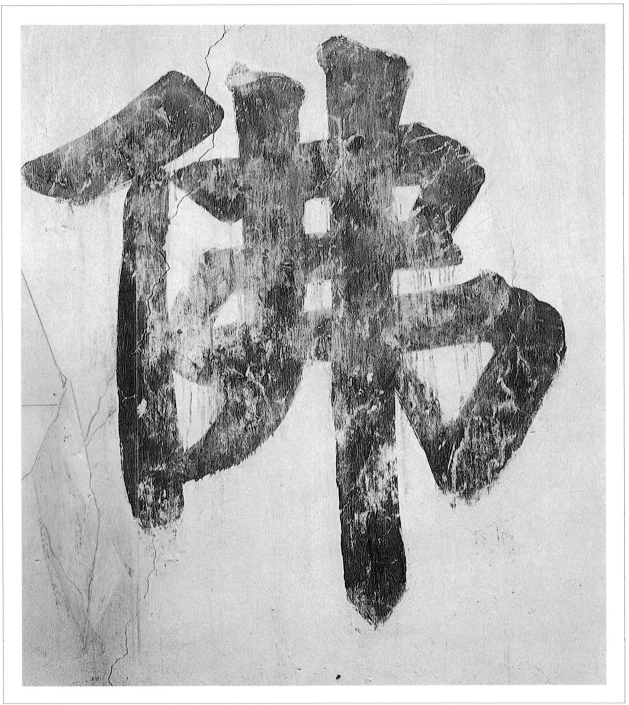

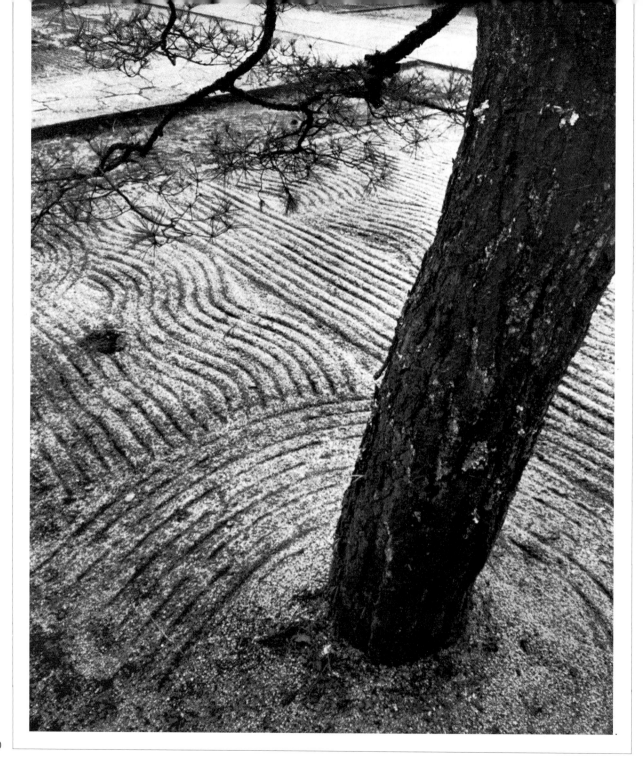

The Foot in the Japanese Tradition

Breathing "from the crown of the head to the soles of the feet."

THE JAPANESE HAVE IMPORTED FROM China, together with acupuncture, some Tao principles in the practice of breathing which center the breath in what they call the "Hara" or "Tanden", which corresponds to the lower abdomen (tanden literally means "cinnabar field" : tan = cinnabar, den = field). Breath originates in Tanden = qi = vital energy.

"... *The reason why concentration on the lower cinnabar field is considered most beneficial is found in the belief that the abdomen is the focal point of the fundamental vital force of human beings. All true primordial energy generated by the practice of Qigong tends to assemble there. The more life-force one has the stronger and healthier one is bound to become.*" [18]

"... *The lower abdomen contracts during exhalation and expands during inhalation . . . All inner organs of the body are greatly stimulated and the digestive and expiatory ailments in particular have been completely eliminated.*" [19]

"... *The cycle of Qi is expanded again to reach from the crown of the head to the soles of the feet during exhalation and back up through the spine during inhalation.*" [20]

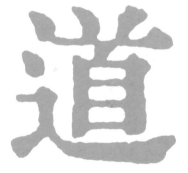

Above: The Japanese imported some Taoist principles and its ideogram, depicted here, from China. The "head" is stylised at the top of the ideogram and the "left foot" is moving forwards at the bottom. In China, the left foot signifies the spiritual side and this Taoist ideogram simbolises the spiritual path.

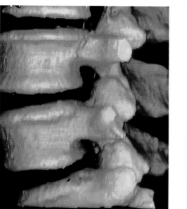 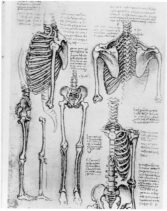

Movements, The Ancient Tradition

W HEN WE CONSIDER MERELY the outer movements of the body, of the torso and limbs, one is astonished at how amazingly simple the exercises are, how easy to perform . . . hardly any effort is necessary . . . So people of any class or age would find them easy to perform.

The movements are essentially stretches of the limbs, especially of the legs and feet. In general, one finds that the feet play an important role in the exercises. In addition there are a certain number of stretches of the back, flexing the torso and swings of the hips. In most cases the movements are undertaken in playful rhythm that ensures that the breathing stays regular and becomes increasingly deeper. [21]

Top left: A three dimensional image of the dorsal view of the human lumbar vertebrae. *Right:* A study of all aspects of the human skeleton by Leonardo da Vinci. *Opposite:* A little girl plays with a hoola-hoop exercising her spine and skeleton playfully, as only children know how to do.

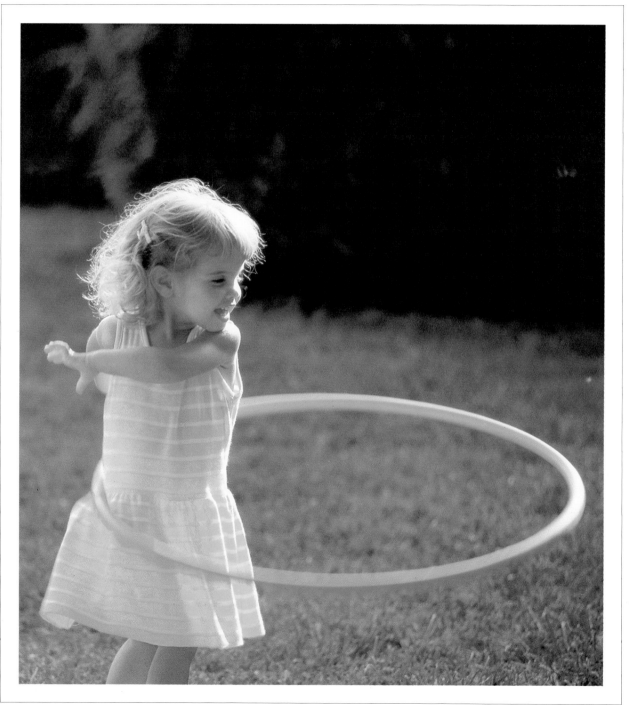

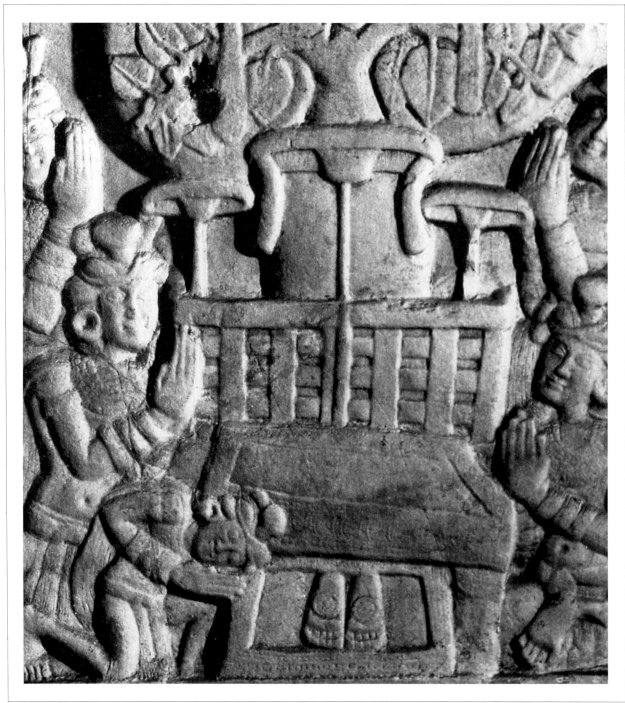

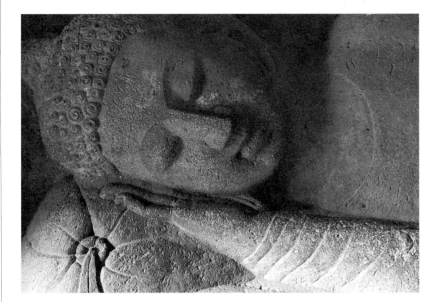

The Foot in the Indian Tradition

THE REVERENCE THAT THE INDIANS HAVE for the feet is well known. To demonstrate their devotion they prostrate in front of their guru or holy person, and kiss the feet.

In the first period after Buddha's death, his figure is not represented in sculptures or paintings – only much later the artists started reproducing the full body.

This photo, taken in Amaravati, in which the Buddha's feet are exposed, shows how his disciples venerated this part of his body. That round wheel on the sole of the feet is called "The Dharma Wheel." It is divided into eight spokes (Eight Spokes Right Fold Path) in which are condensed the Buddha's teachings.

Behind is the stone where he was lying and the tree under which the Buddha received the "illumination".

Opposite: A stone relief showing the imprint of the feet of Buddha in Amaravati, India. A small wheel has been carved in each sole of the foot to draw attention to the Wheel of Dharma, the law of all things.
Above: The head of Buddha resting in his eternal sleep.

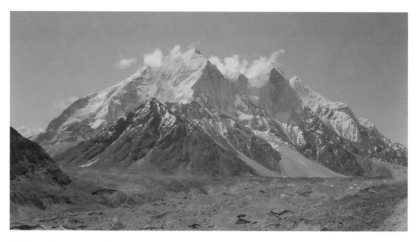

On Attention

Top left: Himalayas, Bahagara Peaks. Their glaciers feed the source of the Ganges.*

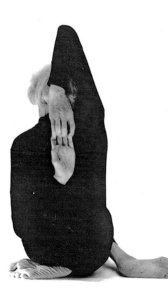

YOGA SHOULD NOT BE A TRAINING for body control; on the contrary, it must bring freedom to the body, all the freedom it needs.

Yoga should help us to acquire the order in the body that it is necessary for it to function properly.

Freedom does not mean license (drink, drugs, smoking, sex), or letting the body fool around with its desires.

Freedom is order in both body and mind. We must give the body clear directions (as we would a horse), and these should be dictated not by ambition, duties or reactions, but by a precise and lucid perception of what we feel. If we are sensitive to the requests of the body, it will respond spontaneously in an unexpected, effortless way. We must create a relationship, make friends with our bodies as well as with our minds.

Freedom is a state of love; there is no love without freedom (Freedom in Sanskrit means love).*

When love is expressed totally through a free, healthy, orderly "body-mind", there is beauty.

* The Sanskrit word for "freedom" is *priya,* from the root *pei,* meaning "to love". Similarly, the word "friend" derives from the Old English freon, which means "to love" (Oxford Dictionary).

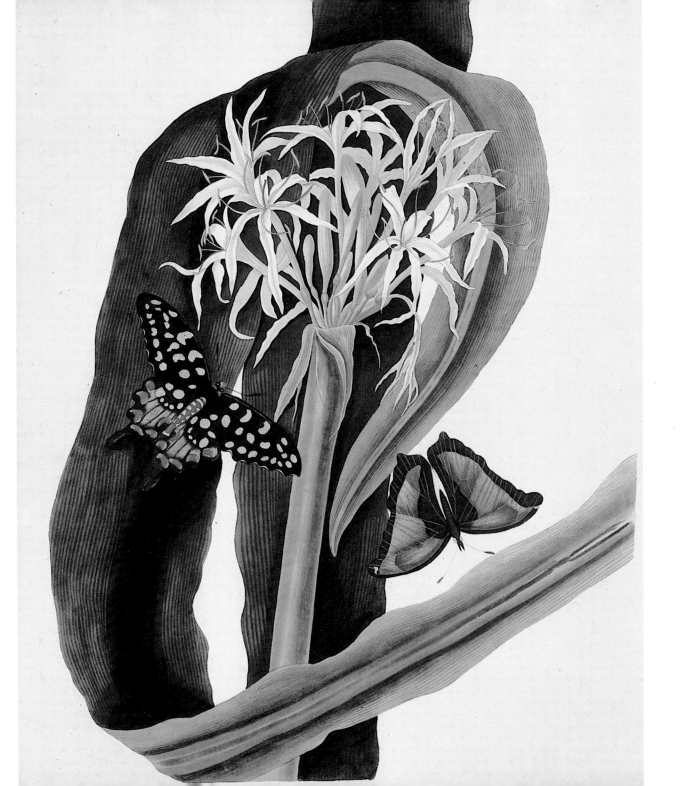

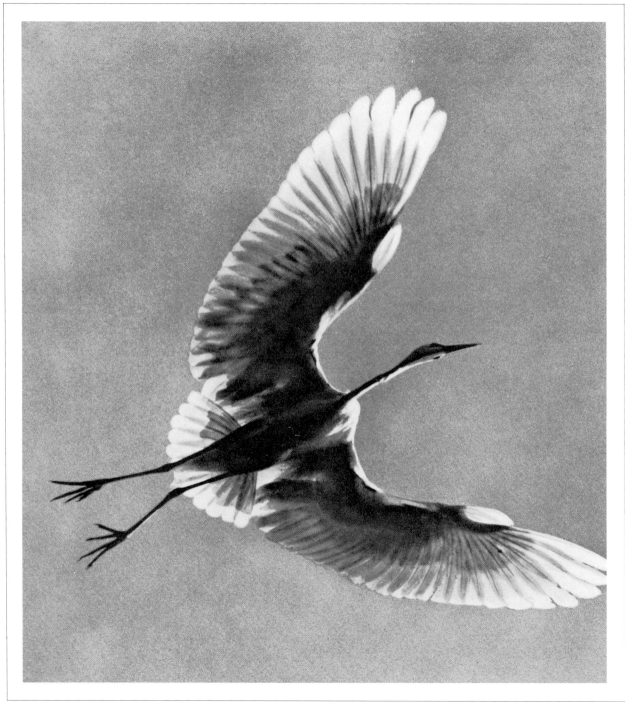

Opposite: An egret, a strong flier, takes off with its long, heavy neck outstretched. Once under way, it will retract the neck into an S and holds its legs stiffly out for balance. To be dominated by fear is like walking between two walls.

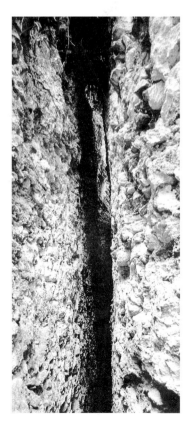

Are you interested in Yoga? (The word Yoga in Sanskrit means union). Are you not curious to discover what happens to your spine, or to your bones, muscles and nerves when you do a pose? What are you feeling when you let gravity take hold of your body? How do your lungs expand during breathing?

We have to completely present in our minds without any distractions. Fear is a distraction from "what is", from the present moment, preventing us from existing, from being what we are.

There is an amusing Indian story that Krishnamurti used to tell to make us understand the state of attention we should have in daily life: *"You must always remember that you live shut up in a closet with a cobra. The moment you are inattentive, the cobra will get you"*.

One has to be extremely attentive and watchful all the time. Such should be our attitude to what happens in us and around us; yet the mind should not be rigid or tied to traditions or patterns, but open and supple, even ready to change direction.

If you know how to "*look*" you will "*see*" that sometimes a disappointment may lead to a new road.

The same happens to the body: if something goes wrong physically, or after an illness, you may discover a different approach or a different perception in the way of doing certain poses, which may even solve other problems. Therefore, do not worry, do not get upset, but keep your eyes and your mind wide open. A disappointment, a loss, may lead you to a liberation.

About Organizations

BE CAREFUL, VERY CAREFUL about organizations.

Yoga cannot be organized, must not be organized.

Organizations kill work.

Love is everywhere, in every thing, *is* everything. But if you confine it, enclose it in a box or in a definite place, it disappears.

When the preoccupations of money, the desire to succeed or the thought of compromise comes into our minds, it is the end.

Yoga is much more serious than all this: it is a living process that changes moment by moment. We have to be with it day and night, feel it in each instant of our existence: watching when we eat, how we eat, when we walk, how we walk, what we say, how we say it. Be conscious of the state of the spine when we sit, of the movement of the brain when we think, why we think, what we think, following our thoughts in operation.

All those things must be present in us and we must be passionately interested in them all.

Truth, like love, cannot be demonstrated, or explained, or offered, it is there with all its immensity around us filling all space. One has only to look. And to be aware.

Here is a good story.

A man was walking along a road, followed by two foreigners. It happened that this man saw something glittering on the path. He picked it up, observed it, and put it in his pocket.

The other two, behind him, saw what he did and one said to the other: "A bad thing for you, isn't it?" But the other man, who was the Devil, answered: "*No, what that man just found is the truth, but I shall help him to organize it*". [22]

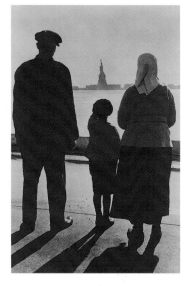

Organizations kill work and cage the freedom of the individual.

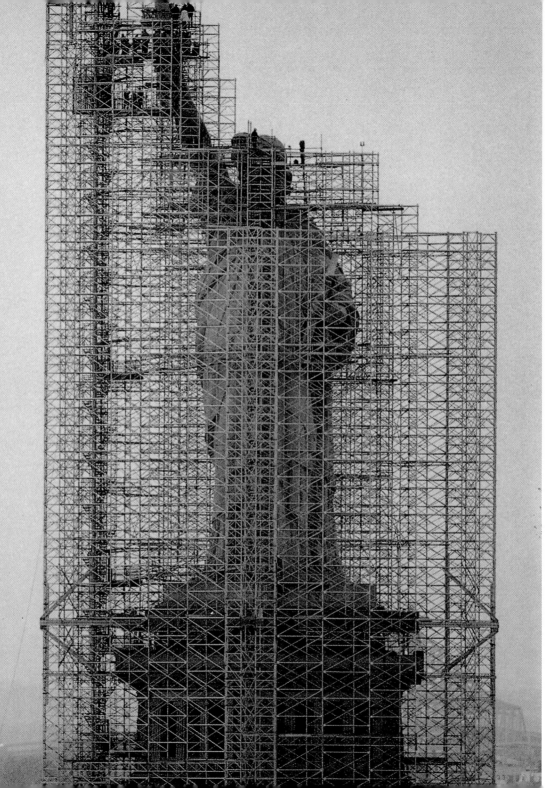

Gravity

WHAT IS GRAVITY — this tremendous force that rules the universe? "*. . . As the force that attracts conglomerates of matter to one another, gravity has a limitless pull. It keeps the moon orbiting the earth, the earth in place around the sun, and our solar system within the galaxy, orchestrating the universe in a cosmic life and death dance*". [23]

"…We are the children of gravity", says Dr. Ralph Pelligra, director of medical research at the National Aeronautics and Space Administration Research Facility in California. "As we age, we reach a point where we begin to yield to it. Sagging skin and organs, varicose veins, arthritis, failing hearts, these all come from the lost battle against gravity."

"*We cannot touch it or see it but it has guided the evolutionary destiny of every plant and animal species and dictated the size and shape of our organs and limbs.*" [24]

Galileo, Newton, Einstein, all worked passionately around this mysterious phenomenon of gravity which holds the miracle of our existence.

Gravity puts us in contact with the spine. All movements we do against the flow of gravity are negative and the ones along the pull of gravity, in which the ground receives our weight, are positive.

While doing the poses correctly, our muscles seem to answer to a binding force collecting them together. This force, responding to the pull of gravity, travels through our limbs and is well accepted by our body, which is always craving for more extension.

We call this force "antiforce". It is similar to the rebounding explosion of a waterfall which, after dropping down at high speed and springing up again with incredible strength (as in the Niagara Falls), transforms and sublimates its journey by dissolving the water into ever lighter sprays creating a swirling cloud.

Opposite: The Niagara Falls. The water is pulled at tremendous speed down the falls, but once it hits the river-bed it springs up again in a swirling cloud. We call this rebounding "antiforce".

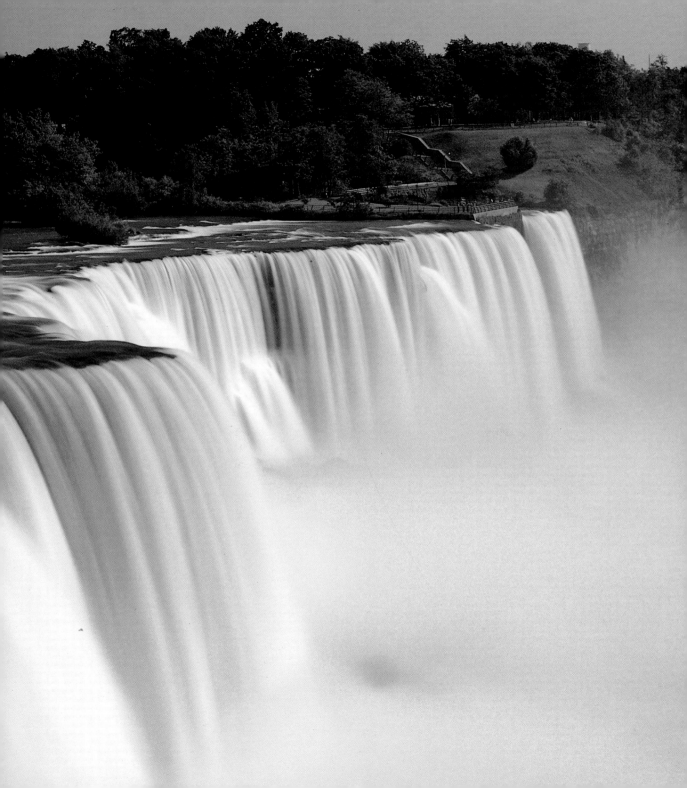

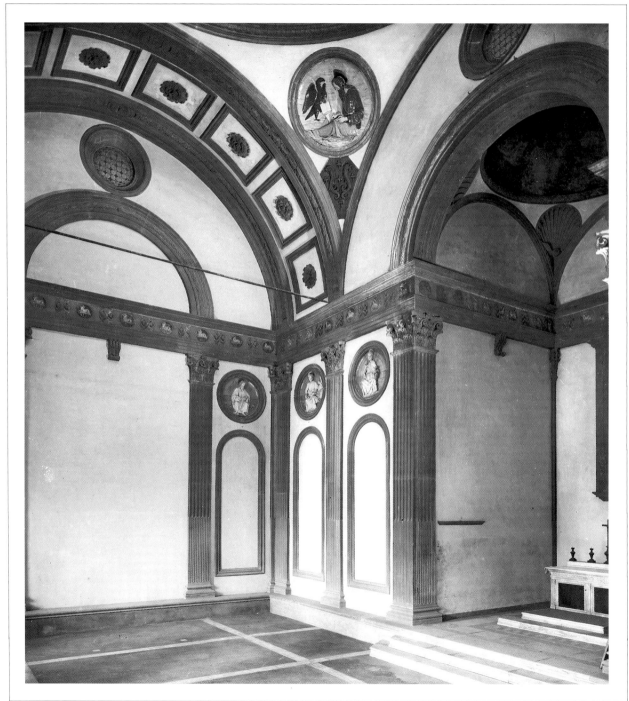

This "antiforce" (= reaction), born from gravity, has its own destiny: the deeper the compression, the greater will be the burst of energy in the opposite direction.

This double movement of force and anti-force, which may sound like a contradiction, operates, with apparent incongruity, also in our bodies: and more precisely, in the waist dividing simultaneously into heaviness (towards the ground) and lightness (towards the sky), obeying a universal physical law. *

The same action is present in the waves of the sea, with that wide extension over the sand and in its rebounding while sucking the water back from the shore.

This also occurs in the projection and reprojection of a sound in an "echo". The sound, reverberating against a wall or against a mountain, is brought back by its own wave.

These reactions are the result of a reflex; a reflex to which our body gladly responds, and which brings about (in a delicate undulatory motion that works like a wave) a healthy, healing renewal.

When the abandonment to gravity comes into action, resistance ceases, fear vanishes, order is regained, nature starts again to function in its natural rhythm and the body is able to blossom fully, allowing the river of life to flow freely through all its parts.

Opposite: Cappella dei Pazzi in the Church of Santa Croce, in Florence, Italy. The chapel was designed by Brunelleschi. The echo in its interior is such that a note produced by a human voice is repeated three times.

* According to Newton's law: "To each action corresponds an equal and opposite reaction". [25]

115

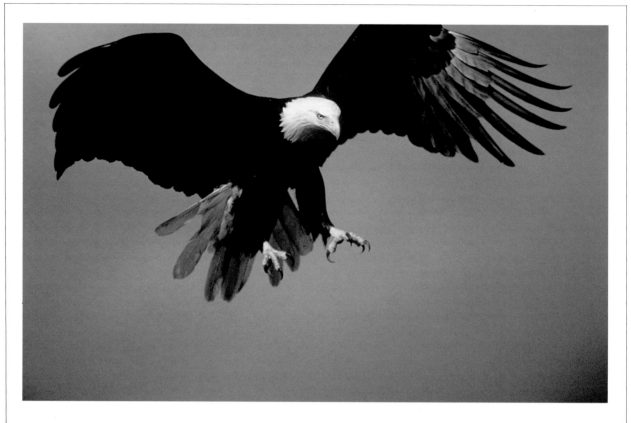

The Eagle

WHEN A BIRD IS LANDING, THE two legs are absolutely straight, towards the point they want to reach (as shown in this photograph of an eagle with its talons touching down on a tree). At the same time its wings are extended to the maximum, they are able to lift so much because the fully extended legs are fully stretched. Again, this dual movement, in two opposite directions, is the result of gravity.

The arms are like wings; we have to learn how to use them. They become light, very light, when the grounding is properly done with gravity under our feet.

Leonardo da Vinci gave a great deal of attention to the flight of birds, since he was experimenting with the possibility of human flight.

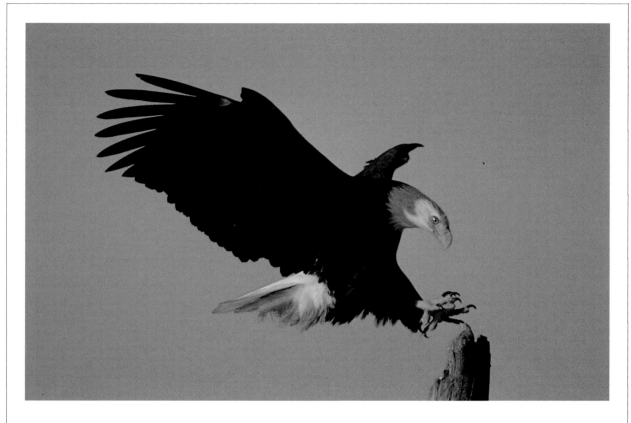

He wrote:

"Quando l'uccello cala, allora il centro di gravità dell'uccello é fuori del centro della sua resistenza…"

("When a bird flies down, then the bird's center of gravity is outside the center of its resistance…")

We must realize that the gravity under our feet, attracting us towards the center or the earth, is outside our bodies.

This is similar to what happens between the earth and the sun. The earth gravitates around the sun, but the sun is outside the earth, attracting it towards itself.

Opposite: A white-headed sea eagle in flight. *This page*: The eagle lands onto a tree-stump. Note the maximum stretch of the legs which point exactly to where the animal is going to land and the outstretched wings. This dual movement is the result of gravity.

117

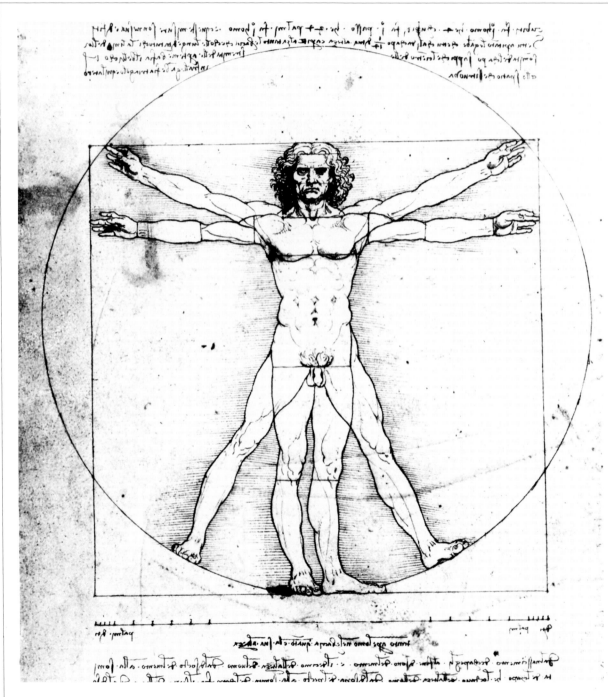

"In the spring of 1505, Leonardo was invited to visit his uncle in the country. During the radiant spring days, Leonardo would stand on the green hill side of Fiesole looking up into the cloudless sky. As he watched the birds soaring in the air, he dreamed of a new type of flying machine. He was also passionately interested in the way the human body was constructed and while Leonardo was in Florence, he dissected many bodies." He studied the position of the bones and where the muscles were attached. He drew the inside section of a skull and made a careful drawing of the heart, under which he wrote, "*A wonderful instrument, the invention of the supreme master*". [27]

As Leonardo examined the marvelous construction of the body, he came to appreciate more and more how precious human life was. "*Let not your rage or malice destroy life — for indeed he who does not value it does not himself deserve it!*" So wrote Leonardo, and from that day till his death he never designed another war machine." [28]

Yoga should help us to protect and maintain our body in good shape, this is an extraordinary gift that was given to us in order to live.

Leonardo da Vinci (1452–1519) was passionately interested in how the human body was constructed. *Opposite*: a famous drawing by the master showing the proportions of the body.

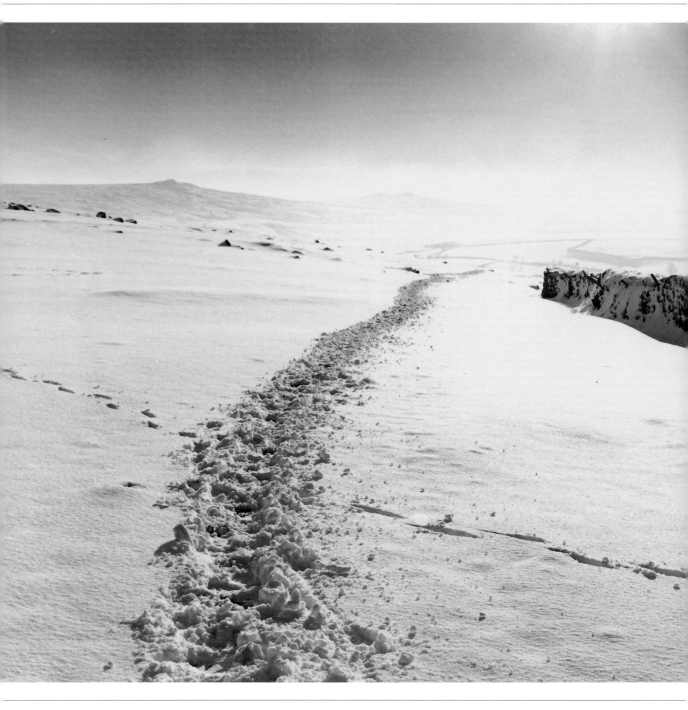

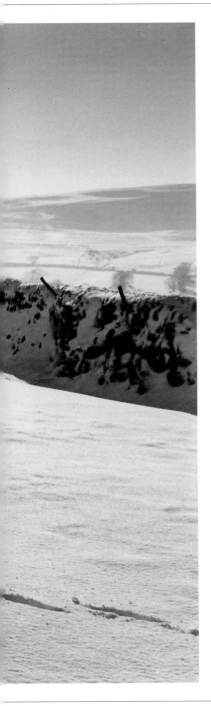

On Walking

CARRY YOUR BODY, but please do not let your body carry you! Walking in the streets, one can see people heavily following their bodies. Their heads leans forwards, pulled by their necks, on their insecure legs, their feet scarcely touching the ground. It is evident that they are slaves to their bodies, following the whispering of their chattering minds.

We must walk well, as animals do.

Put the heels down first placing the feet straight in front of you. Then expand the sole of the foot, allowing it to receive the weight of the body, moving towards the toes. While the other leg moves forwards, continue to keep the back foot on the ground, so that the back of the knee remains extended and open until the last moment before lifting the foot for the next step.

This way of walking will help you to re-establish order, if your body has developed bad habits.

We are always in a hurry, we run, we run, we run, in order to be able to do as many things as possible: to achieve, to become, to obtain. To run is a symptom of fear, to run after something, after somebody. We are slaves not only to others, but to ourselves, to our ideas, to our ambitions, to our projects, and even to our mental projections. This is a miserable attitude that life does not deserve. The slave runs, but the king keeps quiet and remains still in his place.

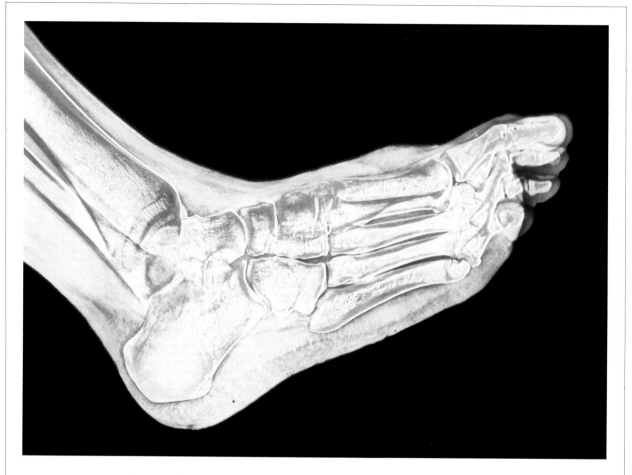

The formation of the arch in the foot is essential in order to stand and walk in a proper way. It can be obtained by directing the weight of the body onto the external part of the heel, keeping it down as long as possible while extending the sole towards the toes.

The picture on this page shows the structure of the foot and one can see the spot at the back of the heel that has to be dropped against the ground and from which the foot should receive the weight of the body pressing the heel forward.

False color X-ray of a human foot seen in side view. The seven small bones which comprise the ankle joint and beginning of the foot are called the tarsus; the large heel bone is known as the calcaneous. The next group of bones (running parallel to the foot) are the metatarsals; these join with the phalanges, the toe bones.

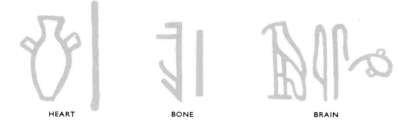

HEART   BONE   BRAIN

These drawings have been copied from an ancient Egyptian papyrus of about 1700 B.C. This ancient medical text indicates that physicians of the time knew something about anatomy. The symbols representing the brain include several phonetic sounds, which presumably indicated the ancient knowledge of the brain as the center of all functions.

The Brain

DID YOU EVER TRY to relax your brain?

The structure of the brain is divided into two parts, right and left.

We can drop the two hemispheres and create space between them. When this happens the two sides will slip aside, like the curtains of a window.

You are then going to discover how much tension was collected there.

Gravity relaxes the brain. This will be possible only if you let the pull of gravity reach the top of your skull.

In this process the many nerves along the channel of the spinal cord will also find relief.

The brain is part of the mind. There must be order in your brain. Avoid the conglomeration of thoughts that brings confusion, and think of one thing at a time.

The mind needs to get clear, logically connected messages from the brain, and, at the same time, it needs to be free to doubt and open to receive and reject all kinds of information.

Surely an open mind is an intelligent mind.

A brain that knows all the answers is a dead brain. From an inquiring, questioning brain arises a healthy curiosity where there will be freedom to explore, freedom to understand, freedom to discover, and in which the looking will be the seeing.

Even the brain needs a rest.

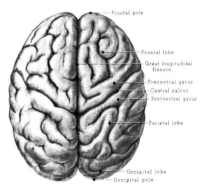

Above: Drawing of the brain with indications of all its parts.

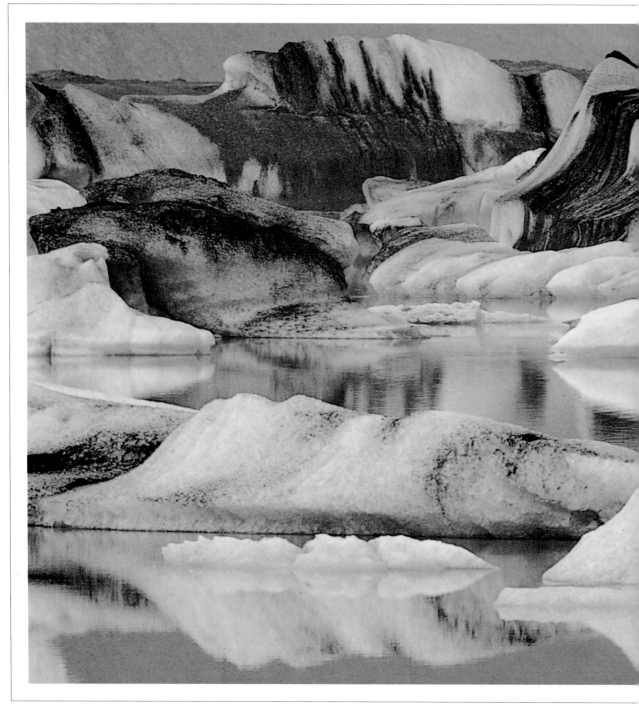

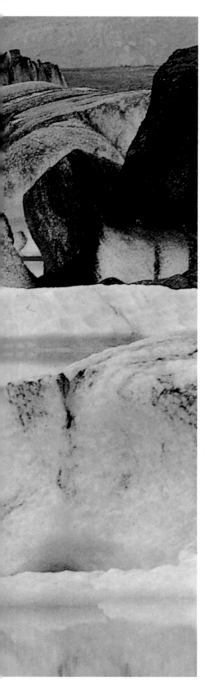

You will be surprised to realize that, when the mechanical section of the brain stops circling around, moving from one thought to another, there will be chance for the brain to relax.

If we can end the swing of thoughts collected by memories in the past, and the ones that have been shaped through fantasy and projected by imagination into the future, we will find silence. Invite silence, welcome silence, and slowly silence will become part of you.

In that silence we will be able to receive hints of intuitions and sparks of perceptions from which creativity can arise.

In Yoga the participation of the brain in the functioning of the body during the asanas is indispensable, as the brain has to watch and follow each movement of the body.

This connection of the brain to the action of the body is a fundamental part of this teaching.

In doing Tai Chi Chuan the body follows the many different patterns of the form. This keeps the attention awakened so that distractions will be avoided enabling the brain to work simultaneously in accordance with the body.

Even when you sit for a while at your desk concentrating on something or finding the solution to a problem, the body, having been restricted, should be allowed to burst out occasionally, reacting with some kind of physical movement. Go for a walk and when you come back you will feel refreshed with new ideas in your thoughts.

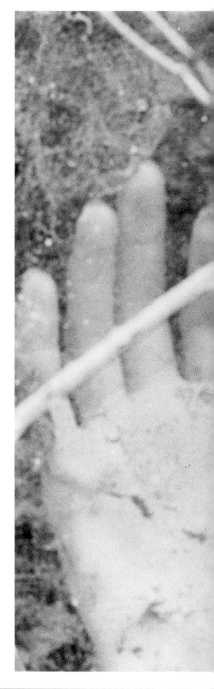

If people only knew how restful it is for the mind to be with "what is!" All that running away from the present is tiresome, useless and leads to mediocrity.

The adherence and contact with what is going on in the present moment is a healthy state of awareness. And the communion with nature around us, or with any other human being or situation, is part of our existence.

When the unnecessary, and even harmful, struggle of "becoming" that leads only to mediocrity stops, one "is" and the immature grasping along the ladder of ambition disappears.

Reasoning is connected with the brain, but intelligence functions within the mind.

Mathematicians and philosophers, such as Aristotle, Descartes, Kant and so many others, follow the laws of logic, trying to keep in tune with a severe pattern that will satisfy the brain but will not satisfy the mind. The mind needs another element to function totally, as the rational pattern is not adequate to its demands. What is this request? Is it passion? Is it love?

Is it that element of unification, beyond the limits of thought, where body, brain and intelligence come together, opening the communication with that vast immensity in which mind and universe meet?

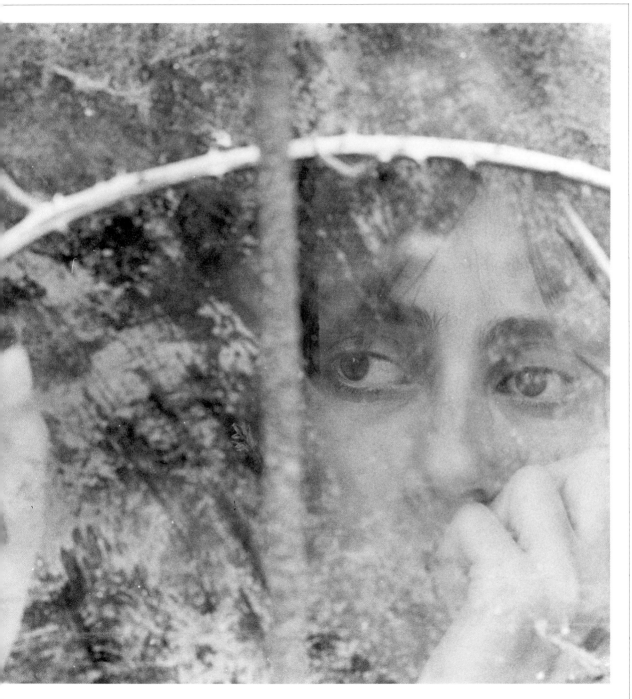

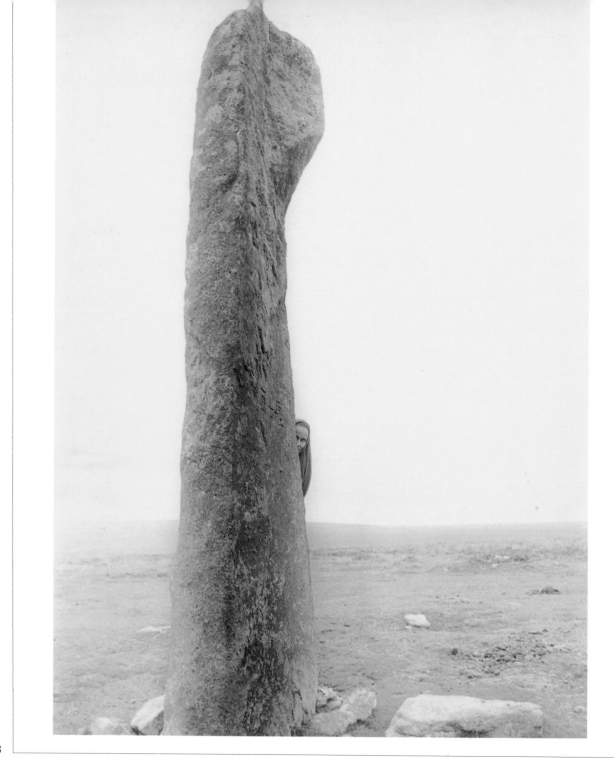

A Meeting with Death

TO BE ALONE IS TO BE with everybody, with everything. Avoiding people or running after things leads to isolation.

To accept the one and to reject the others is to be exclusive.

To resist, to withdraw, to depend is a consequence of fear. Fear of what?

We defend our possessions against others, we are afraid to lose them, to be invaded. We hold to illusions, ideas, ideals. After all, when we die we leave everything and when we arrive in this world we have nothing. Why make so much fuss about it?

Let us be simple, let us follow things without sticking to them.

A very well-known Italian poet, Gabriele D'Annunzio said: "Io ho quel che ho donato." – I have what I have given.

And here is another well known story, this time from the Orient:

Death meets a servant in the market and announces to him that in three days he will come to take him away.

As soon as Death disappears, the servant, desperately afraid, goes to his master and with broken words and broken heart tells him about this strange meeting and asks him for a horse so that, running as soon as possible and as far as possible, he can go to a distant place and avoid Death.

His Master, feeling terribly sorry for him, answers: "You have been a faithful servant, you have worked many years for me accomplishing your duty with devotion and intelligence. Do take my best horse, the one that can run the fastest, and go, leave at once. Fly away."

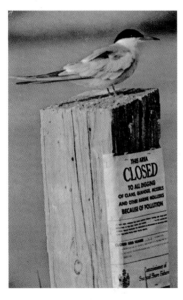

Opposite: The fear of death and solitude may be caused by an unconscious regret of not having loved or given enough. *Above*: The freedom of a small bird unaware of written regulations imposed upon humans.

The servant thanks his master, goes to the stable, chooses a lovely Arab horse and leaves, riding the animal as quickly as he can.

For three days and three nights, without stopping, he travels to escape from Death, he runs, and runs, and runs.

At last he arrives at Samarkand, and feeling safer and far enough away, sees a nice garden and stops to take a rest.

Right there he is greatly astonished to find Death again.

Death, coming slowly towards him, says:

"I was so surprised to find you at the market three days ago, in that distant town, because I was supposed to meet you here today and take you away from here."

We cannot escape from our destiny and we cannot avoid death.

Why are we running so much? To die earlier? Why do we resist death?

It is an unconscious hidden regret because we feel that our possibilities to love have not been totally accomplished? We could have given more, we could have loved more.

Let us be less impatient. Let us be more wise and take things easy.

If the āsanas are done peacefully, this yoga will indirectly slow us down (also improving the immune system which suffers from stress) and strip us out from many useless and harmful efforts, giving us the feeling of a different quality and introducing a delicate fragrance into each day's existence.

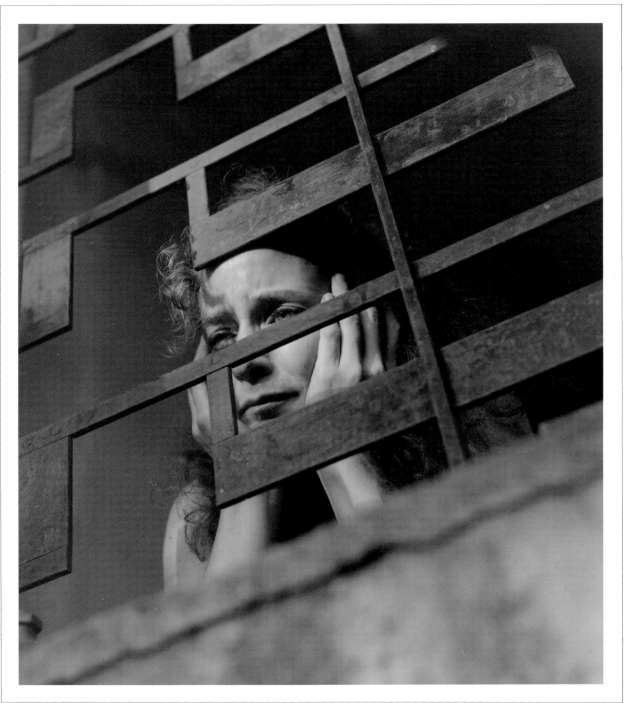

The Necessity of an Empty Mind

TO BE PROUD OF OUR YOGA POSITIONS is bad taste. To be able to do the poses "successfully" means nothing, nothing at all. Yoga should not become a circus. It must not be done as a refuge from life.

Though yoga will somehow protect you, it cannot be *used* to protect, or *made* to give health.

It should instead help us to purify the body and the mind bringing us back to that blessed state of receptivity from which we can start to learn.

A Zen story tells of Nan-in, a Japanese master, during the Meiji era, who received a university professor. The professor came to inquire about Zen. Nan-in served tea. He poured his visitor's cup full, and kept on pouring. The professor watched the overflow until he could no longer restrain himself.

"*It is overfull. No more will go in!*"

"*Like this cup*" Nan-in said, "*you are full of your own opinions and speculations. How can I show you Zen unless you first empty your cup?*"

"*. . . Suzuki Roshi . . . told his students that it is not difficult to attain enlightenment, but it is difficult to keep a beginner's mind.*" He told them: "*there are many possibilities, but in the expert there are few*".

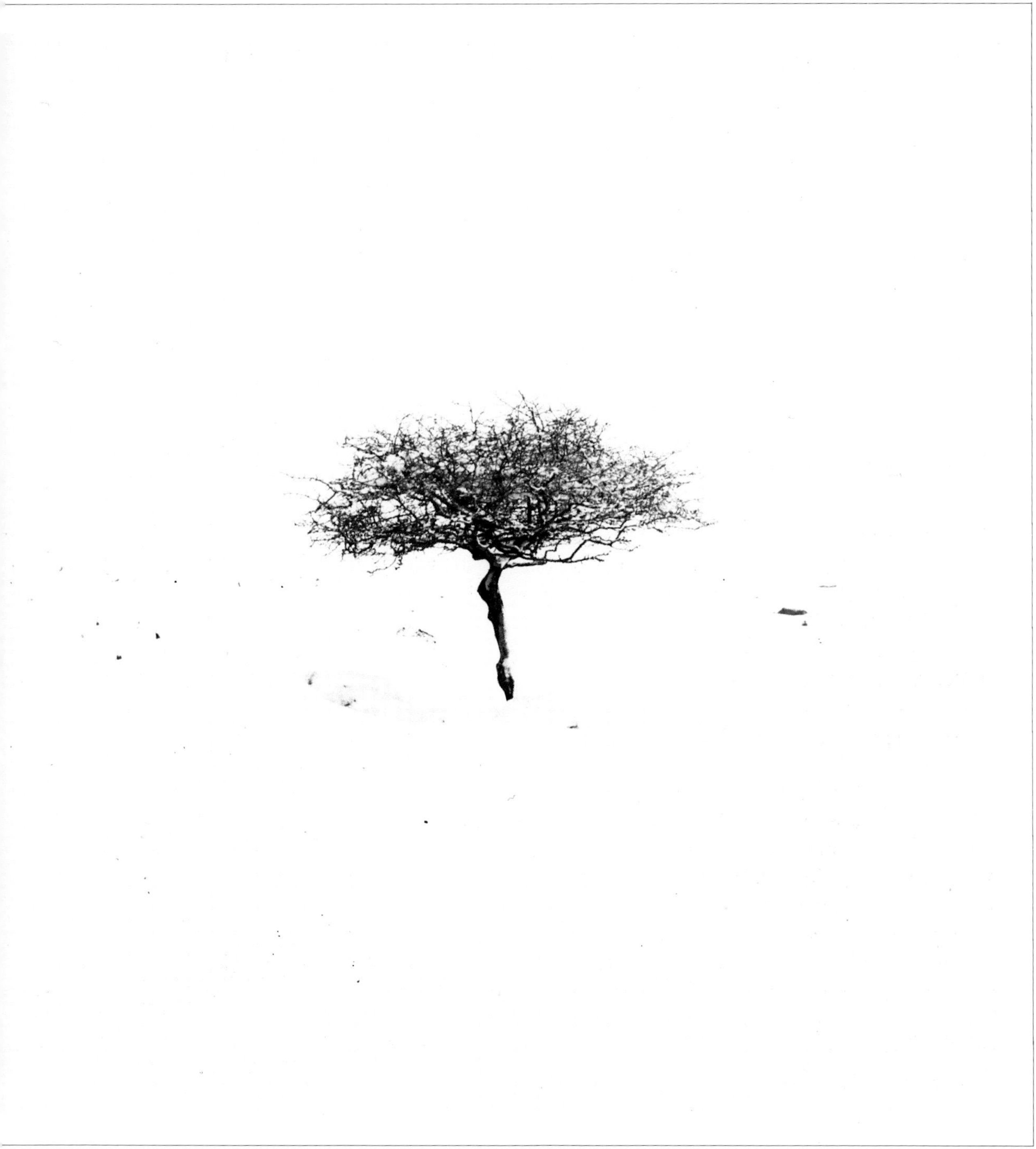

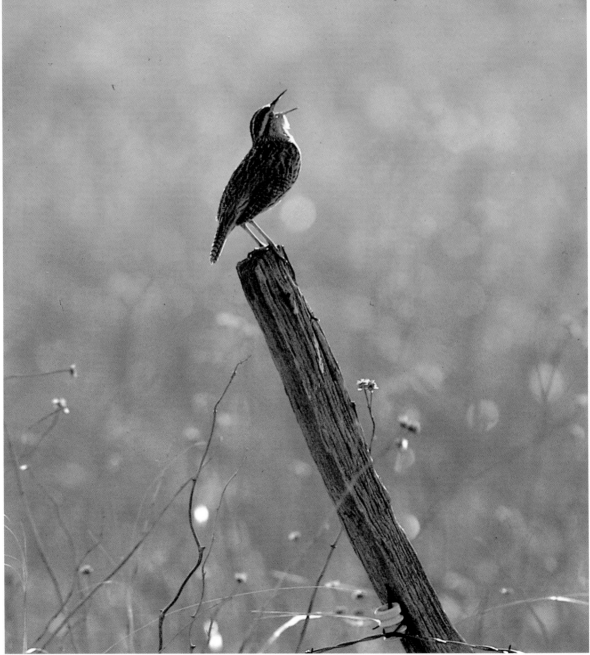

When his students published Suzuki's talks, after his death, they called the book, appropriately, "*Zen Mind, Beginner's Mind*". In the introduction Baker Roshi, an American Zen master, wrote: "*The mind of the beginner is empty, free of the habit of the expert, ready to accept, to doubt, and open to all the possibilities . . . .*" [29]

Yoga could also give us the possibility to create space (between one action and another action, between a breath and another breath, between a thought and another thought) allowing emptiness to inundate our minds, as Leopardi says in that beautiful poem – "L'infinito":

"*Così tra questa Immensità s'annega il pensier mio: E il naufragar m'è dolce in questo mare*".

("And in this immensity my thought is drowned and it is delightful for me to be shipwrecked in this sea").

Therefore keep your body relaxed, sensitive, awake and your mind fully alert, watchful, while observing.

Perhaps something unexpected will come to you, it might come from quite a different or even opposite direction.

Sometimes strange things happen, let us be open to receive them.

"*Once a Zen master just set down to pronounce a sermon, when outside a bird started to sing. The master did not say a word and everybody listened to it.*

When the bird stopped singing the master simply announced that the sermon was over, and he moved away". [30]

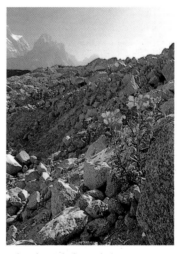

A lovely pink flower, the only survivor after the storm. True creativity and alertness only arise when emptiness has seized the mind. *Opposite*: a meadow lark giving a masterly sermon with a song.

Practical Suggestions

Opposite: a scene of rural delight. Contact with nature slows one down and ordinary activities can become a source of immense pleasure.

WHEN YOU WORK IN YOUR GARDEN or while you do weeding, as you bend forwards, if possible keep your knees locked.

When you wash dishes, remain with your stomach close to the sink and do not let it stick out. Keep standing on your heels.

When you wait in a queue, keep your feet straight in front of you in contact with the ground, and your back erect. Do not let your head lean forward, keep your chin in and rely on your heels.

While driving, if you are alone, breathe regularly. If it rains, breathe to the rhythm of the wind-screen wipers as they go back and forth (like a clock marking the seconds). You will remain independant of your car's acceleration and your heart rate will not increase when the speed increases.

When you eat, do not eat in a hurry, but eat slowly, relaxed and chewing long (salivation being indispensable for a good digestion). It is not so much *what* you eat as *how* you eat. You are going to discover that you eat less, as your stomach will not be so anxious to receive food. Eating in a rush is also the cause of many stomach troubles.

A hard bed is better for the joints and especially for the spine. If possible, sleep without a pillow, so that the neck can rest naturally. When using a pillow the neck is curved for hours at unnatural angles and will not be able to relax properly.

While watching television, sit comfortably but keep the back straight. If you cannot sit in "padmāsana" (cross-legged), you can sit on your heels, or in any other position as long as your back remains erect.

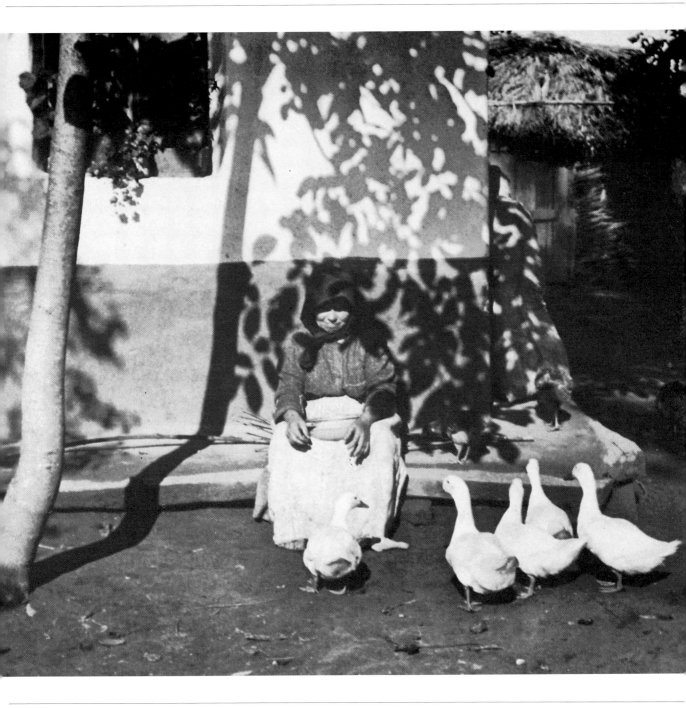

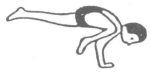
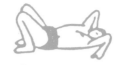

The Advantages of Doing Yoga

YOUR EVERYDAY ACTIVITIES WILL improve and become more efficient. You will have less time for useless occupations, that are constantly in the way, preventing your contact with more essential things. It is like a sieve through which superficial things drop away leaving only what is essential.

You are going to have a better digestion if you do some poses before eating when you are tired.

You will need to sleep fewer hours, as your body will be more relaxed during the night.

You will gain a few inches, eliminating that curve along the back of your spine, and therefore you are going to be a little taller.

You will be able to stand for hours without getting tired, if you gravitate properly on your heels with the knees straight.

You will be able to improve the poses, as there is no end to progress.

You are going to straighten yourself if one part of the body is weaker than the other, by paying a lot of attention while doing your poses, and by continuing this attention throughout the day you will reach a better balance.

You will no longer be a slave to your body, as the independence from it is the greatest gift you can receive.

Health is freedom. When we are healthy the body is not "in the way", it will be better prepared to react against illness and disease.

The presence of the body should not be felt negatively. It is only when it does not work properly or when it is ill that we feel

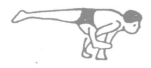
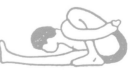

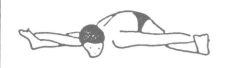
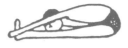
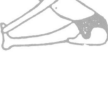

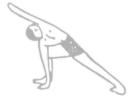

encumbered by its presence. Even when a small part of it is disturbed (like a mild pain in a cut finger; or a simple cold that blocks your nose, keeping you busy the whole day with a hankerchief in your hand; or a sore-throat which makes you lose your voice), it heavily reminds you of its existence and you are obliged to become conscious of it all the time.

Yoga is a way of life, it changes you and therefore changes the way you relate to other people and influence your environment.

As the sun opens the flowers delicately, unfolding them little by little, so the yoga exercises and breathing open the body during a slow and careful training.

When the body is open, the heart is open. There is a transformation in the body's cells. They work in a different way and a new growth is possible.

What is that binding force that holds the many worlds together and with its intensity also attracts us to each other? Can we call it Gravity, Energy, Love?

Dante Alighieri closes his famous poem *"La Divina Commedia"* with these words: *"L'Amour che muove il sole e l'altre stelle." "Love that moves the sun and the other stars."* [24]

To re-establish contact with our body is to be in contact with Nature, is to be in contact with the Cosmos.

Balance is restored, space is around us and that tremendous power, arising from the earth in unison with these universal forces, will become part of us.

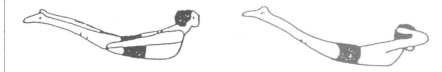

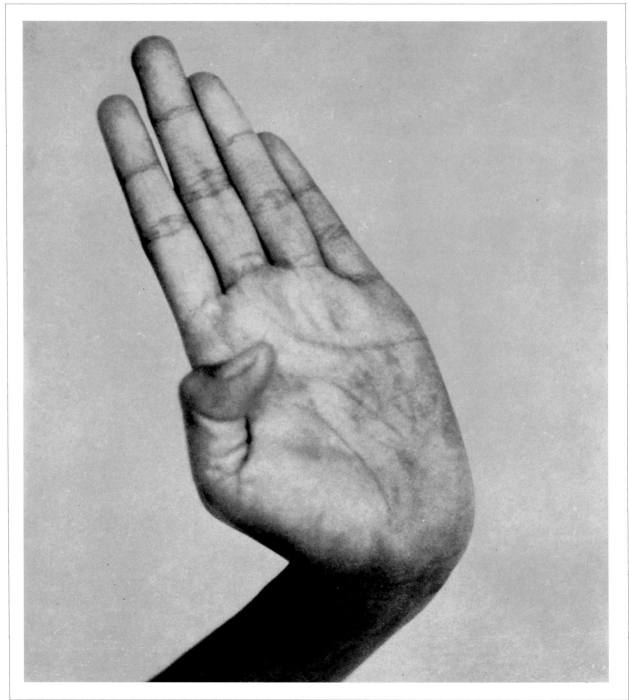

Part II

The Ãsanas

Tadasana – Utthita Trikonasana – Utthita Parsvakonasana – Virabhadrasana – Parivritta Trikonasana – Utthita Hasta Padangustasana – Sirsasana – Halasana – Salamba Sarvangasana – Supta Trivikranasana – Bakasana – Supta Vajrasana – Bhujangasana – Urdhva Dhanurasana – Kurmasana – Suptakurmasana – Adu Muka Svanasana – Marichyasana – Andra Mastyendrasana – Pasasana – Malasana – Kandasana – Mulabandasana – Viranchyasana – Yoga Nidrasana – Kapotasana – Eka Pada Rajakapotasana – Eka Pada Viparita – Natarajasana.

The Āsanas

ERE ARE JUST A FEW of the many poses of Yoga. Perhaps following the explanations for each exercise will help clarify one or two points for both the beginner and the more accomplished student. They are offered, in any event, to make their practice more interesting, more attractive and even more beautiful.

I was encouraged to write this book to help my pupils discover the beauty that in this work becomes "art" when it is handled with the right approach.

These photographs of a few Āsanas portraying Vanda Scaravelli and some of her pupils, do not correspond to a formal, orthodox or acrobatic pattern, but are meant only to show that the poses can be done in an agreeable, supple, relaxed and natural way.

Tādāsana *(Mountain pose).*

This is the most important pose. Do it right and all the others will follow.

In Tadāsana the body is perfectly still.

Standing on the back of the heels your weight slowly sinks down. If you stand long enough, while the lower part of the body, from the waist to the heels, gravitates, you will discover that the upper part of the body becomes light, free and straight. This starting position can correct and adjust spinal problems such as scoliosis, arthritis, lordosis, etc.

To do the pose correctly stand on the back of the heels with the spine straight, knees extended and chin in. The weight must be distributed equally on both legs.

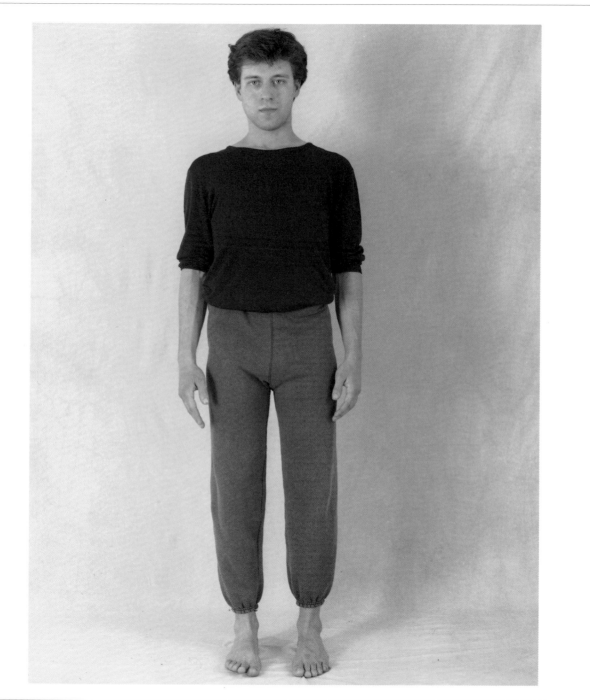

Utthita Trikonasāna, Utthita Pārsvakonāsana, Vīrabhadrāsana, Parivritta Trikonāsana, Parivritta Pāsvakonāsana.

These standing poses are entirely based on the heels. The weight of the whole body falls on the back leg. Keep the heel of that leg solidly on the floor and allow the other parts of the body to be loose and light. Do not let your arm drop towards the floor until the body is completely turned, then the twist is over, and you have only to bend.

Vīrabhadrāsana

These poses are the same as the others, with the weight of the body mostly on the back leg and heel. While bending forwards, to balance, you are lifting the back foot all the time and there is an extension in it. While rising, the foot in the air, try to roll it gently in.

Utthita Hasta Pādāngusthāsana

As in Virbhadrāsana, in this pose, convey the weight to the foot that is on the floor, making it heavy, very heavy, while the other one in the air becomes light and easily lifted.

Top, from left to right: Utthita Trikonāsana, Utthita Parsvakonāsana, Utthita Hasta Padangusthāsana. *Bottom, from left to right*: Parivritta Trikonāsana, Virabhadrāsana. *Opposite*: Virabhadrāsana.

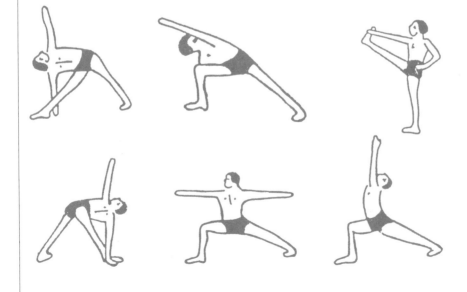

144

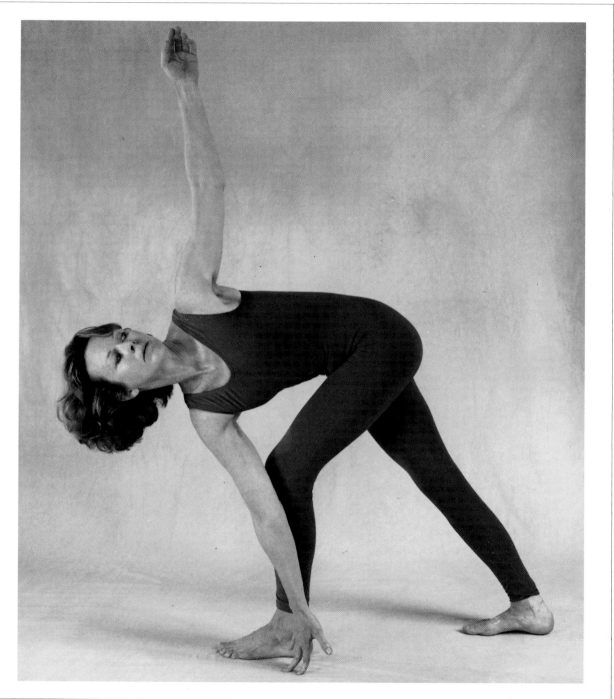

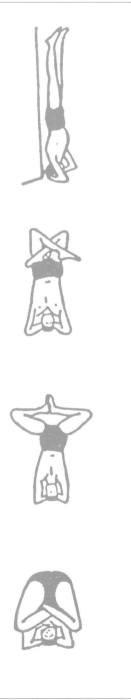

Left, from top to bottom: Salamba Sirsāsana, Urhdva Padma Sirsāsana, Buddha Konāsana, Pindāsana in Sirsāsana. *Opposite*: Front and side view of Sirsāsana.

Sīrsāsana *(Headstand)*

This position is the cause of many cervical distortions and arthritis. These disabilities arise from the way people lift up with the chin out allowing the weight of the body to fall on the twisted neck. This gives the pose a wrong start.

To avoid this mistake you should do the preparation before lifting against the wall, or even better against a corner, keep the knees bent close to the eyes, and the chin down towards the chest (chin lock), the back of the head adhering to the wall (or the corner), pulling elbows down until the legs move naturally and easily up, not with a jump.

In holding the pose, during each exhalation, keep the elbows down, traveling from the elbows towards the wrists, pressing elbows and wrists on the floor and bringing slowly the weight of the body towards the head. Extend the knees from the elbows (sinking the elbows into the floor). Let the lumbar region gently touch the wall (or the corner).

There must be life not only in the front part of the body but also in the back part of it.

Often one side of the body (generally, in the right handed the left side) is weaker, therefore one must give attention to it, making the leg, hip, shoulder and wrist on the left side more efficient, twisting them towards the center.

During these poses keep your eyes wide open so that you can correct the "āsana" if the head is not straight and legs are not in line and parallel. Perhaps a mirror will help.

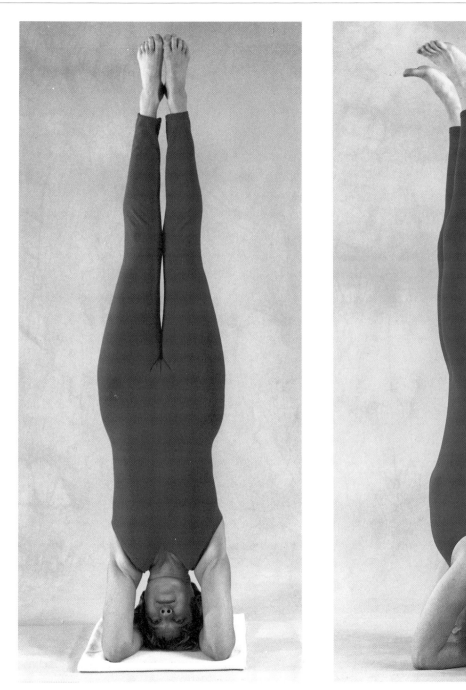

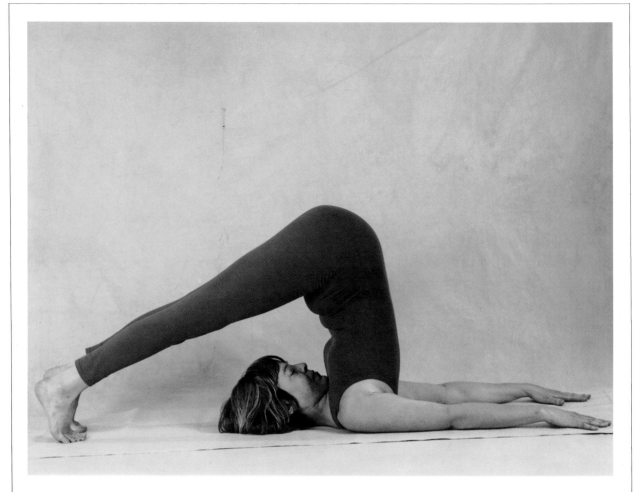

Above: Halāsana. *Opposite, left*: Parsvaikapada Sarvangāsana, *middle*: Ekapada Sarvangāsana, *right*: Salamba Sarvangāsana.

Halāsana (*Plough Pose*)

Lie down before raising your body vertically up in Sarvangāsana (shoulderstand) and extend your legs over the head with knees straight (elongating the inner part of the knees). Keep hands with palms on the floor. Roll the wrists extending them slowly towards the fingers.

Sālamba Sarvāngāsana *(Shoulder stand)*

While still in Halāsana bend the arms towards you and support your back with the palms of your hands. Then lift the legs up. Lean comfortably on your arms, with the elbows down elongate the spine, bringing the weight of the body towards the shoulders (remember that it is called Shoulder Stand), and stretch your knees. Press the elbows on the floor each time you exhale, keep the knees locked.

The legs become light and rise freely (because of the inversion of gravity). The body should be absolutely in line (as in the head stand). Often one side of our body is stronger than the other, this is why many people hurt themselves. One should learn to adjust the two sides of the body equally and evenly, as well as keeping the head straight. Letting your chin drop into that little hole, between the collar bones at the base of the neck, will help you to put your head right.

From the shoulder stand go back into the plough pose, touching the floor with your feet. Then, keeping your head on the floor, and making your body heavy and relaxed, roll your spine down along the floor, and feel it massaging your back. Watch carefully that both your legs reach the ground perfectly in line.

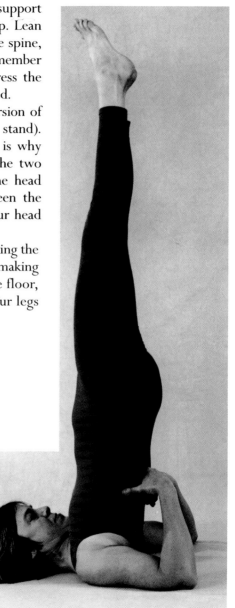

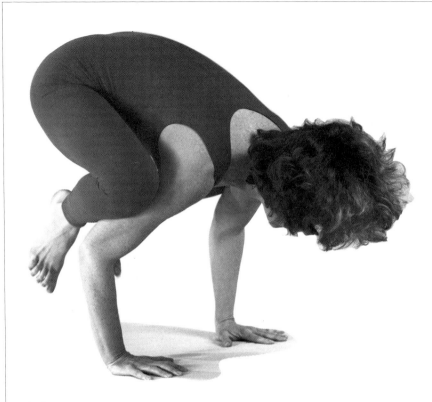

Left: Bakāsana. *Below, from top to bottom*: Bakāsana, Parsva Bakāsana. *Opposite*: side views of Supta Trivrikramāsana, *below*: Anantāsana and Supta Trivrikramāsana.

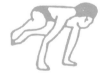

Bakāsana (*Balancing pose*)

Before lifting, balance your body with hands on the floor and knees bent under your upper arms. Extend the palms of the hands on the floor, pressing the wrists towards the fingers and relax arms and shoulders.

Tuck in your legs around your arms.

Bring all the weight of the body over the hands discharging the head from its load (one cannot lift the head, if the head is heavy). This will help you to come up easily. While lifting up press the wrists down towards the floor in the direction of the fingers, and keep the elbows backwards so that the body will be pulled in two opposite directions. This double movement of the arms, formed by the wrists forwards and the elbows backwards, is very important.

While holding the pose follow the flow of the balance and drop your bottom as if you would sit on the floor.

This exercise and its variations are particularly good for the liver.

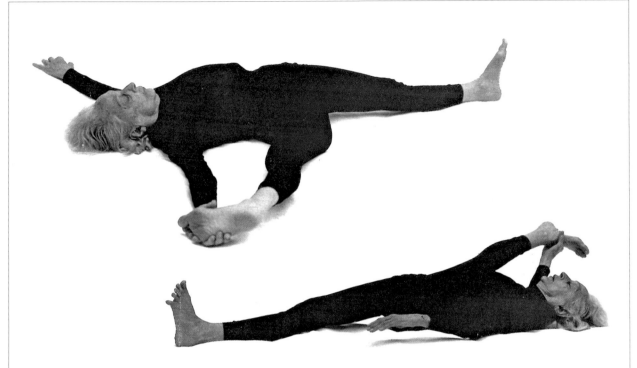

Supta Pādāngusthāsana *(One leg up, one leg down)*

In this pose, while exhaling, before lifting your leg up, you must elongate the opposite leg down on the floor extending the knee. Do not pull the upper leg with the hands but the movement has to come from the spine.

Elongate your spine, touching the floor with the back of your waist, this pressure will make the more distant parts of your body (the head and the feet) lift a bit. It is like the two opposite ends of a "gondola" curling and turning up its bow and stern.

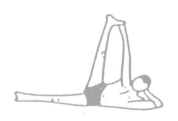

To extend the upper leg out to one side touching the floor, lift the leg up first with knees locked turning it towards the ground, lowering it in little round movements. Do not force or push it down without lifting it first.

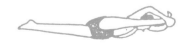

Advantages: In the extension of the back, the spine elongates and the abdominal muscles work.

151

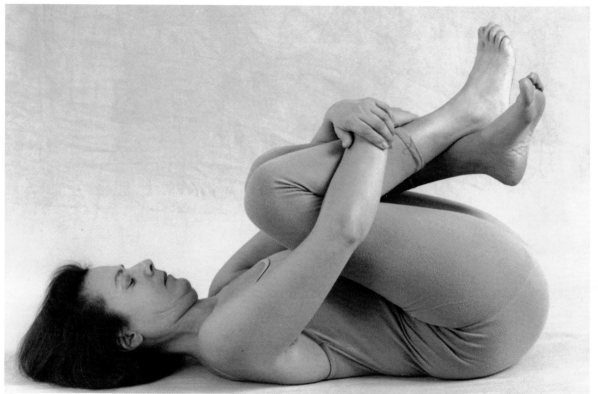

Supta Vajrāsana (*Little boat*)

Above: Supta Vajrāsana.

Lie down with knees bent, feet on the floor. There should be no curves along the spine (if you bend the knees with heels on the floor it will be easier). You will be able to find out if there is a hollow along the spine by putting an arm under your waist. If there is still space there, while exhaling keep pressing the spine against the floor until it is completely flat.

Then lift your legs with bent knees towards your chest, keeping your arms around your legs and with them press the body against the floor so that the spine, and especially the waist, will come in contact with the ground (as shown in the photograph). And you can swing agreeably from right to left as a little boat. Exhale peacefully all the time.

Advantages: This movement will strengthen the abdominal muscles that are generally weak.

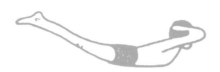 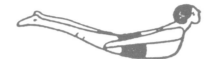

Salabhāsana (*Simple back-bending*)

These poses should prepare the spine for the back-bending. They are very interesting and should be done with understanding and great precision, the movement centering in the spine.

Lie down on your stomach, feel the movement of your spine with each breath and follow its wave from the very bottom of it, in its extension.

Lift the upper part of the body from the floor a little, rising very slowly from the spine. Do not push forwards with the head (the head remains relaxed and loose following the ascending elongation).

The movement of the spine in these three poses is similar: it must originate from the base of the spine, travel all along the spinal vertebrae reaching the neck and behind the skull, giving life to the spinal cord. This unblocking of the vertebrae is a delicate journey and needs to be watched with attentive care.

Do not bend at the waist (remember the waist must elongate) or lift from the arms, but lift only from the spine, pressing the muscles of the thighs against the floor (this will extend the waist in the lower part of the spine). Arms are loose and head is light following the spinal movement.

Inhalation and especially exhalation will put life into your spine.

Bhujaṅgāsana (*Cobra pose*)

Do this exercise only after you have worked on the previous three poses (simple back-bending) for some time, because to hold the āsana from the legs and hips (without restricting the spine on the waist) needs a good deal of tightness in the thighs, therefore one has to wait until those muscles are formed and ready to perform the pose.

In the Cobra pose the lifting is stronger and one can hurt oneself if it is not done perfectly as has been explained in the three previous āsanas. Done correctly it should not damage the spine.

Below: Bhujaṅgāsana. Opposite Urdhva Dhanurāsana.

Urdhva Dhanurāsana (*Back bend from the floor*)

Lie down on your back with knees bent, feet on the floor and arms extended over your head, your chin in.

Elongate your spine while exhaling slowly and happily.

Touch the back of the waist to the ground (like in the little boat).

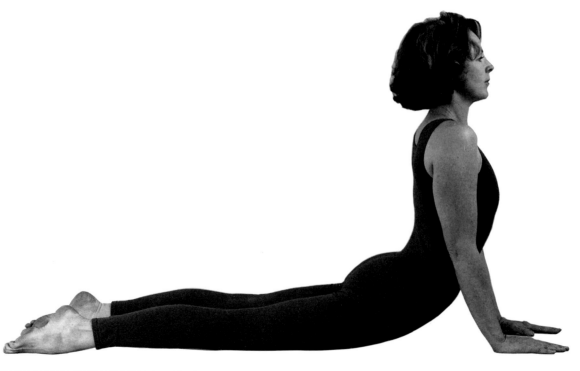

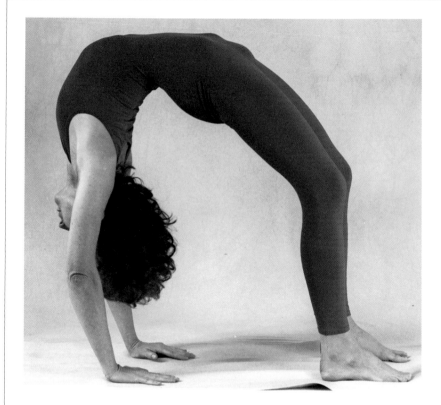

Put your hands on the floor close to your shoulders, bending your elbows and turning them slightly inwards as if they had to touch each other, letting them circle in a slow round movement towards the center, drawing little circles in the air (like rowing in a boat).

This is going to relax your shoulders and send the weight of the body towards the feet.

Make your hips heavy and large.

Let the soles of your feet extend and spread (the toes remain light and are able to lift) Let the heels sink down. Do not resist gravity. Like a magnet it pulls the feet vertically downwards towards the center of the earth. Focus your attention on your heels, keep all your waist touching the floor, and with exhalation rise up, keeping your chin in.

Pushing up to Urdhva Dhanurāsana.

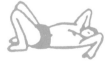

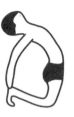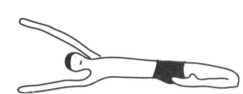

Top, from left to right: three preparations for backbending, chest-shoulder stretch; chest-abdomen stretch; abdomen stretch. *Below*: going down into Urdhva Dhanurāsana. *Opposite*: Urdhva Dhanurāsana, backbending against the wall.

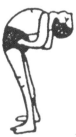

Urdhva Dhanurasana (*Back-bend from standing*)

This is the most important and one of the most difficult of the yoga poses. It implies the total lengthening of the spine from the heels to the head and it requires a great deal of attention.

This re-awakening of the spine is going to give you a new flow of vitality and, if it is well done, a new vigor will fill your body.

Stand on your two feet like in Tadāsana.

Let the gravity of the earth take hold of your body. Heels (and especially the back of the heels) are gravitating deeply downwards.

The soles of the feet remain in contact with the ground, as if there was glue under them.

The knees are locked by the pulling of the heels.

The muscles of your thighs become firm.

The outside of the legs, from the hips to the little toes, turn inwards (as if they wanted to reconstruct the figure of the skeleton).

The whole of the legs, like two solid columns, hold down the lower part of the body (from the waist down). At the same time the upper part of the body (from the waist up) is becoming lighter and lighter lifting all the time vertically towards the ceiling (in the opposite direction) therefore it is easy to bend back dropping the upper part of the body towards to the floor.

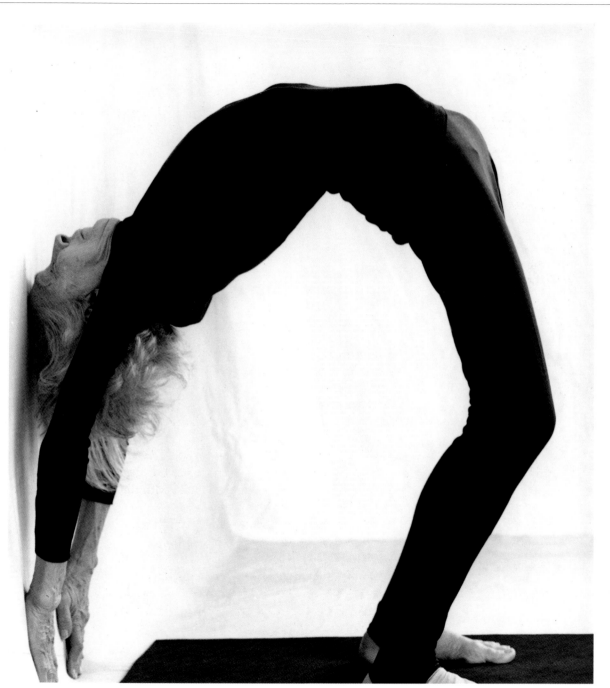

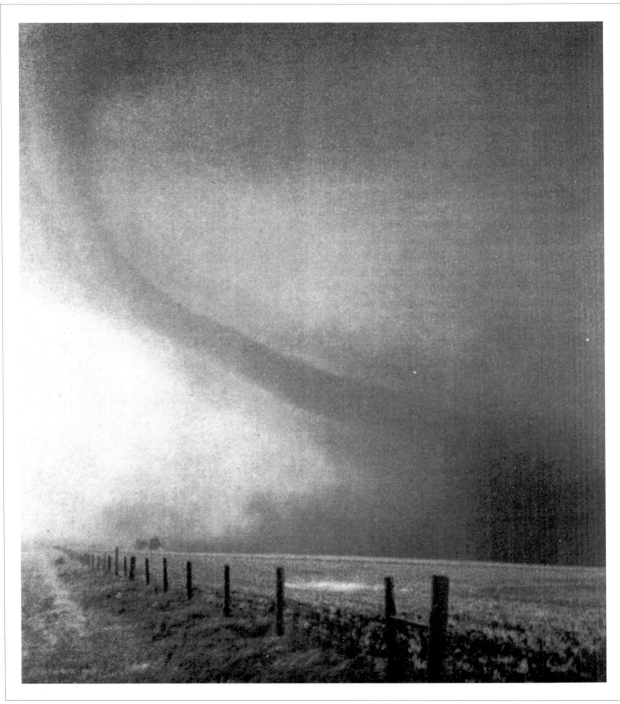

Following the wave of breathing, each exhalation brings us — simultaneously lower (from the waist down) and higher (from the waist up) in a double movement (your chin should remain in) with the eyes looking straight ahead.

One must not fall on the ground, but, as we can observe in the photograph, the body is controlled until the end by the elongation of the spine and especially by the elongation of the last vertebrae.

We could compare this movement to a whirlwind that, after having sucked and turned the water violently downwards into an eddy vortex at tremendous speed, then lifts the massive conglomeration of water high up into the air, collecting it in a single column and rejecting it down into the sea once more.

In essence the same thing should happen to the body: gravity, in taking hold of our heels and legs, pulls them downward, like in a vortex, bringing lightness to the upper part of the body — curling, rejecting, and reversing our trunk in the opposite direction.

The stronger the sucking, the higher and suppler the elongation of the spine toward the sky and the deeper its rebounding to the floor.

"... There is the image of the spiral movement which represents the "tornado" (Robinet 1979: 169-183), a curled power that created the world and moves in alternating motions of advance and retreat. The image of the spiraling wind unifies the two main concepts of time, irreversibly linear and eternally cyclical, and simultaneously contains a steady upward motion of ascent. It is at the same time a curve that bends back onto itself and a route that leads to even further progress..."[25]

Gravity takes hold of our legs and heels and at the same time brings lightness to the upper part of the body, like the movement within a vortex.

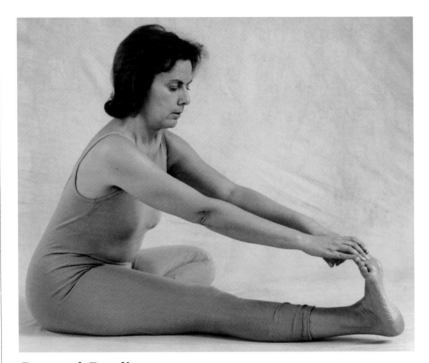

Forward-Bending.

The movement we have to do in the forward-bending is similar to the one we do in the back bends. Only the trunk bends in the opposite direction – foreward instead of backwards.

While exhaling, the lower part of the back of the spine, from the waist down (and in particular the three last lumbar vertebrae) should drop towards the floor *before* bending. Such action will give lightness and flexibility to the upper part of the spine. This part will lift spontaneously and therefore bend easily. Never bend without lifting first. It is an agreeable motion similar to the wave in the sea rising up and dropping, splashing on the shore. It gives elasticity to the whole of your back, making it more supple and free. There is such happiness in this undulation!

Most of the forward-bends, through the wave movement of the spine (rooted in gravity) are projected in the horizontal direction.

Above: Maha Mudra. *Opposite*: *top*, Prasarita Padottāsana; *bottom*, Upavistha Konāsana.

160

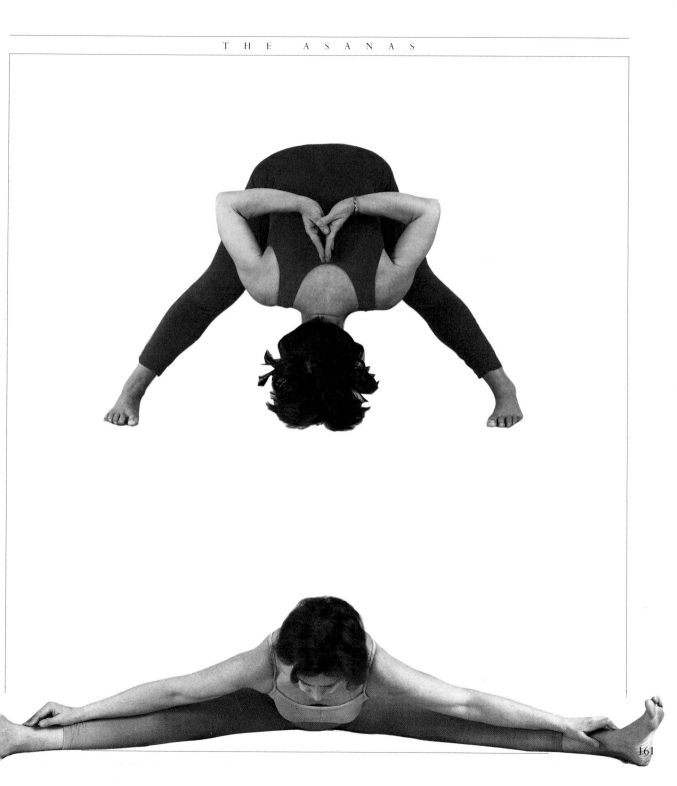

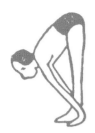

Uttānāsana

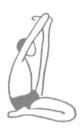

Krounchāsana

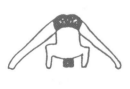

Prasarita
Padottānāsana

To move from the spine implies a total movement from the center (the spine) to the periphery (the extremities), or, as one might say, from the body outward (to the external). Instead, when we move from the extremities it is a partial, peripheral movement (from the external towards the body), which causes strain.

Along the pull of gravity the muscles (through the spine) work correctly, lengthening and elongating outwardly, in an unlimited fashion, in the right direction (from in to out).

Instead, when we contract incorrectly, restrict, or squeeze the muscles, moving inwards from the periphery (from out to in) they shorten, limiting us. This indicates that the direction is wrong. Thus we find ourselves pushed into a corner.

To put it in another way:

In contrast with the powerful gravitational flow which comes from nowhere and goes far away, there is the brutal aggressive force obtained by the compression of the muscles. It has very little run (being confined to a definite point) and is generally used against a person or an object. Your breath shortens and you become exhausted.

This is the substantial difference between these two opposite actions. We have to get a clear idea not only about the vertical pull and flow of energy, but also about the horizontal line. Both depend on gravity. Both are connected with the spine and centered on the spine. Let us play together with it. Ask someone to bend your arm. Your muscles contract to resist, but if the pull of the other's pressure is strong, he will be able to bend it.

Now let us try it working in the right way:

Stand on your heels, gravitate down, lean slightly forwards with one arm straight in front of you. Imagine your arm is in a large tube, wrapped in energy, as if it were drawn by a rope, traveling along that horizontal line, slowly pulled without limits in that direction. Your arm becomes like iron and nobody will be able to bend it.

Another experiment that can be done, this one along the vertical line, is about the weight.

Stand firm, but not stiff, on your feet, heels and legs, while you receive the load of your body, and let the gravitational pull reach your whole person, as if you had to sink in the depths of the earth. If you are without resistance your body will become heavier and heavier, the dropping will be immediate and powerful, and it will be almost impossible for someone to lift you.

Uttānāsana *(Forward-bending)*

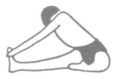

Mahā Mudra

In this Asana the only thing you have to do is to let your heels gravitate deeply down and stretch the knees from the heels. This will elongate the upper part of your body, giving elasticity to the spine. Do not lean back, but keep the trunk forward and arms relaxed and loose.

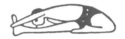

Janu Sirsāsana

Prasārita Padottanāsāna

Keep the back of your heels down bringing the weight to the external part of your feet. Press together the palms of your hands behind the back.

Krounchāsana

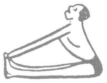

Bend the elbows and bring the feet to the head and not the head to the feet. The head must remain still, in its place and receive the feet.

Mahā Mudrā

This is one of the most complete and efficient exercises. Knees and legs get extended from your hands, the shoulders drop and become straight, the back of the spine elongates, the belly is drawn inside, the chin is pulled towards the neck, and the head will easily find its right position.

Paschimottānāsana

Jānu Sīrsāsana, Paschimottānāsana, Upavishta Konāsana

If the pull of gravity is properly achieved in these three poses, Janu Sirsasana, Paschimottanasana and Upavistha Konasana, by keeping the lowest part of the spine gravitating deeply on the ground, you will discover that the two parts of your spine will gain distance from each other. One feels as though a drawer opens in the middle of your back. This will untie and loosen the upper part of your body.

Upavistha Konāsana

163

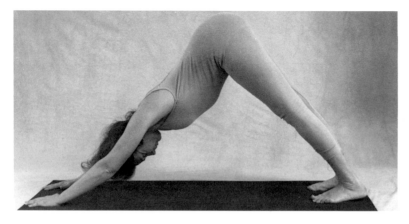

Adho Mukha Svānāsana *(Dog-pose)*

In the dog pose the only movement that should be done is from the ankles pushing both heels towards the floor.

The more you elongate the ankles towards the ground, the more the shoulders will benefit. The spine straightens and becomes supple.

Elongate the spine walking like a dog (keeping on the spot) with alternate legs and hands.

Gallop like a horse by pulling down heels and hands at the same time (keeping on the spot).

After all quadruped animals are elongating their spine at each step. We are less lucky.

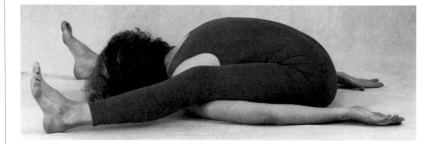

Kūrmāsana

Sit with legs straight in front of you.

Put your arms underneath the legs and then under your thighs, and stretch your knees by pushing your heels forwards.

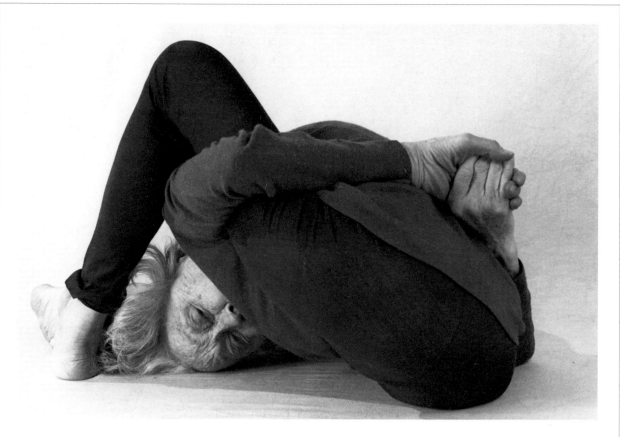

Elongate your spine.

Touch the floor with your forehead and after more extension you will be able even to touch your chin with your face flat on the floor.

Supta Kūrmāsana *(Tortoise)*

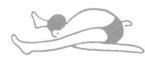

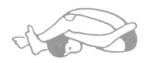

Go into Kūrmāsana

Then bring your arms back closer to your body and with the elbows on the direction of the floor extend them towards the hips.

Reverse the hands on your back with the palms up, bend the elbows and lift the hands until they catch each other.

Bend your knees, bring your feet closer to your body and cross them at the ankles. Put your head in that inviting little space between your feet and your knees that, like a nest, receives it and gives you a rest. Breathe and relax.

Twists

The three twists described below should each be preceded by leaning the body forwards and elongating the arm, which needs to be wrapped around the bent knee. Bend the elbow (as close as possible to the ground) as if you wanted to touch the floor with it.

Marīchyāsana

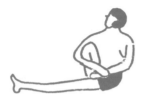

Sit on the front of your foot with one leg bent and the other straight in front of you, with the opposite arm around your bent knee.

Bend completely forward on your toes making a long arm outside your bent knee.

Go back very slowly until your heel touches the floor, while remaining with your body bent as forward as possible.

This will create interesting opposite movements.

Then catch your hands and lift from the spine.

Ardha Matsyendrāsana

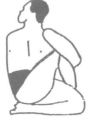

Sit on the arch of your foot (half padmāsana – lotus pose). Cross one leg over the other with the knee bent and the foot on the floor. Bend forward with the arm outside the opposite knee and extend the arm. Make a long arm and, with your elbow bent, creating space and turning ribs and stomach aside. Catch the other hands behind your back, sitting on the arch of your foot and lift the spine up, pressing the other foot on the ground.

Pasāsana

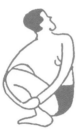

While squatting, bend knees forward with feet on the ground. Stretch one arm forward to the maximum. Bend it around your knee and keep your elbow as low as possible trying to touch the floor with it. Bring the other arm across the highest part of your back and catch hands.

Double movement: Elbows down forwards and heels back on the floor.

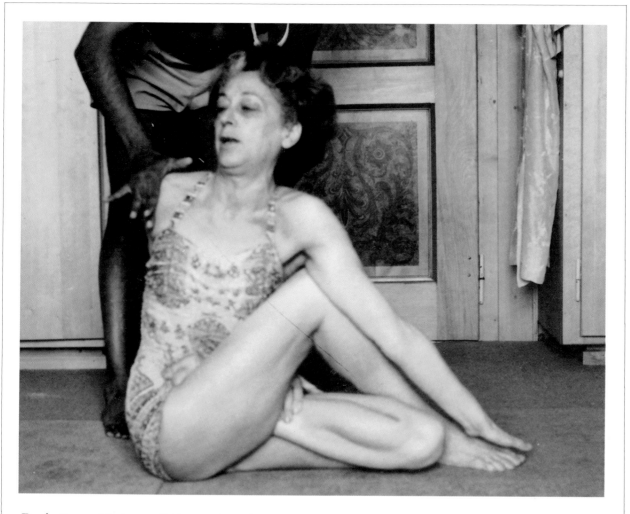

Paripūrna Matsyendrāsana *(Double twist)*

Sit on the floor with knees wide open, spread out directly in front of you.

Put your hands under the external part of your feet making the soles meet. Slowly, bring them as close to your body as possible until they touch it.

The knees may be a little high during breathing, most noticably while exhaling. Do not be impatient for while it takes time they eventually will descend to the floor.

Above: Paripurna Matsyendrāsana.

Left, top to bottom: Marichyāsana, Ardha Matsyendrāsana, Pasāsana.

Malāsana

Squat forwards with arms bent, turned inside along your hips and thighs, into the inner part of your knees. Try to touch the floor with your heels. Keep one elbow as low as possible towards the ground. Turn your hands back, reversing the palms up, lift them a little and bring them together.

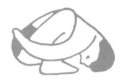

Left: Buddhakonāsana. *Middle*: Mūlabandhāsana. *Above*: Malāsana.

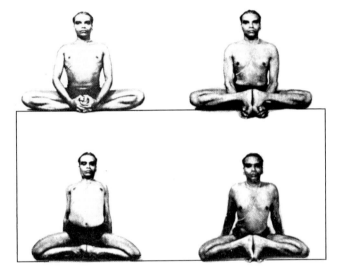

Left: Mūlabandhāsana. *Middle*: Mūlabandhāsana. *Above*: Kandāsana.

Kandāsana

Sit as shown in photograph (Buddhakonāsana) with knees touching the floor and both feet on the floor near your body.

With your hands turn the soles of your feet upwards reversing them completely. Press the outsides of the feet together, where the little toes are, touch nails with nails exposing the soles, as if you opened a book and read it, and lift them slowly turning the front of your feet inside. Keep knees on the floor and breathe.

Bend your arms bringing the palms of your hands together in front of you, let them meet in the way of an "Indian salute" ("namaste") and keep still.

The space between the palms of the hands is called "Angeli" in Sanskrit.

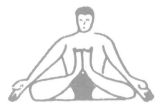

Mulabandhāsana

This pose is an exceptional and difficult Āsana that very few are able to do without damaging their knees as it entails the inversion of the ankles and heels. One should not teach it. It is shown here only for the fun of it.

Sit on your knees with toes back and heels in front of you. Spread your knees little by little, separating them until reaching a straight line.

Slowly push your heels forward. Keep hands over the knees. Bring your body always further back towards the toes. While breathing in this pose, a hole will be formed in your abdomen.

The advantage of doing this exercise is that the muscles of the abdomen are pulled and drawn inside, causing even the last vertebrae of the spine to elongate.

Below: Vanda Scaravelli in the pose Mulabandhāsana.

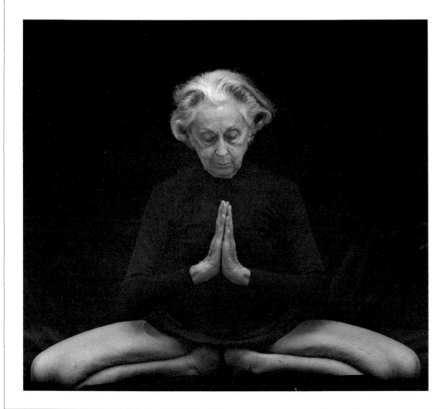

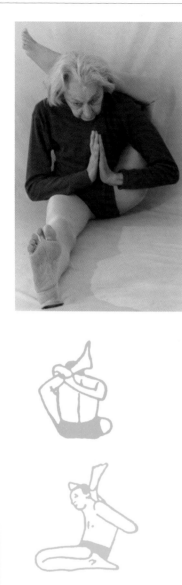

Viranchyāsana

Sit on the floor with one knee bent and take the other foot and ankle in your hands trying to bring them up behind your neck (it should be even lower behind your shoulder).

While lifting your leg, roll it gently in small little circles. Do not push, but wave it with care. Take time.

Kapotāsana (*Back-bend with knees bent on the floor*)

Kneel down with arms up loose behind your shoulders. Do not bend backwards until you feel that the knees are planted in the ground and that your hips are gravitating deeply and solidly on the floor.

The muscles of the thighs should be strong enough to sustain the body while the reverse wave takes place, rising vertically up and consequently down. (Do not bend from the waist, but from the lower part of the spine). Because of the pulling down of the thighs, the upper part of the body becomes light and will be able to lift easily. Exhale naturally each time you lift in order to bend in a pleasant, effortless way. Keep your chin in with your eyes looking towards the ceiling and drop on the floor with elegance.

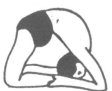

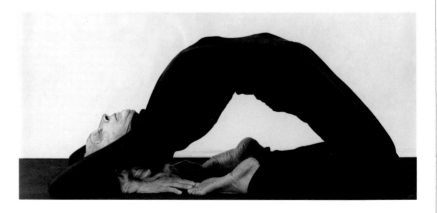

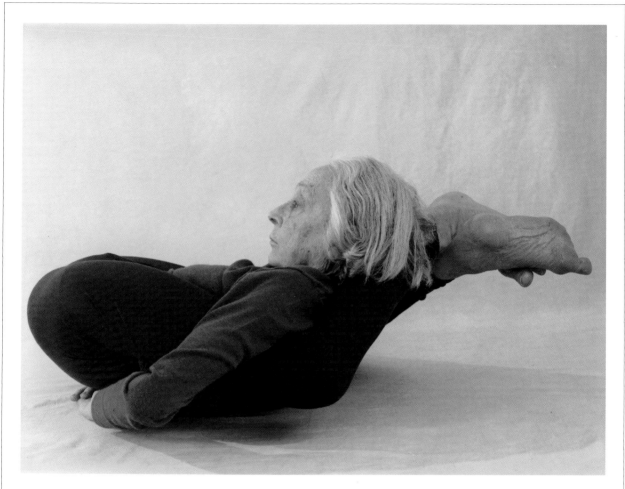

Yoga Nidrāsana (*Yoga sleeping pose*)

Go into Halasana (plough pose), bend your knees and delicately bring your your legs one after the other behind your neck. Tuck in the ankles at the base of your head behind your skull: This is the cushion where the yogi puts his head when sleeping in the position. From there drop forward into the Yoga sleeping pose.

Draw your hands behind your back with the wrists on the floor and let them catch behind your waist. Take a good rest.

Left: Top; front, back and side view of Viranchyāsana. *Bottom:* Kapotāsana. *Above:* Yoga Nidrāsana.

171

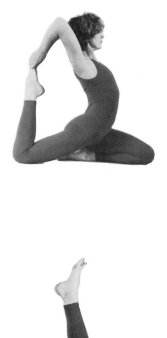

Eka Pāda Rajakapotāsana

First go into Hanumañasana, or complete leg split.

Then bend the front leg in the half lotus pose (with the knee on the floor) and lift up the back leg (bending at the knee). With a lot of care slowly catch your back foot with both hands. Loosen the shoulders, elongate the spine, keep your head free and breathe regularly.

Eka Pāda Viparita *(Back-bend on elbows with one leg up)*

Bend your knees on the floor, kneeling, and extend the lower part of your arms forward in front of you.

Elbows, arms and hands are solidly and firmly on the floor, while the elbows move towards the wrists.

Lift your legs up.

Bend the knees, lifting them higher and higher as if you wanted to touch the ceiling with them before letting them drop down on the floor.

Lift one leg vertically up straight, pointing to the ceiling, pressing the other one on the ground. Lift your head from the floor. Catch your ankle with your hands, if possible.

Natarājāsana

Stand absolutely firmly on one leg with the roots digging well into the ground (knees locked).

Lift and bend the opposite arm on the back over your shoulder letting the hand to catch the foot on the same side. Extend now the other arm straight in front of you (the one on the same side of the foot on the floor).

Do not bend at the waist, on the contrary, extend the waist creating space and bend, instead, on your thighs, pushing them down.

The beauty of this pose is in the freedom and lightness of the upper part of the body.

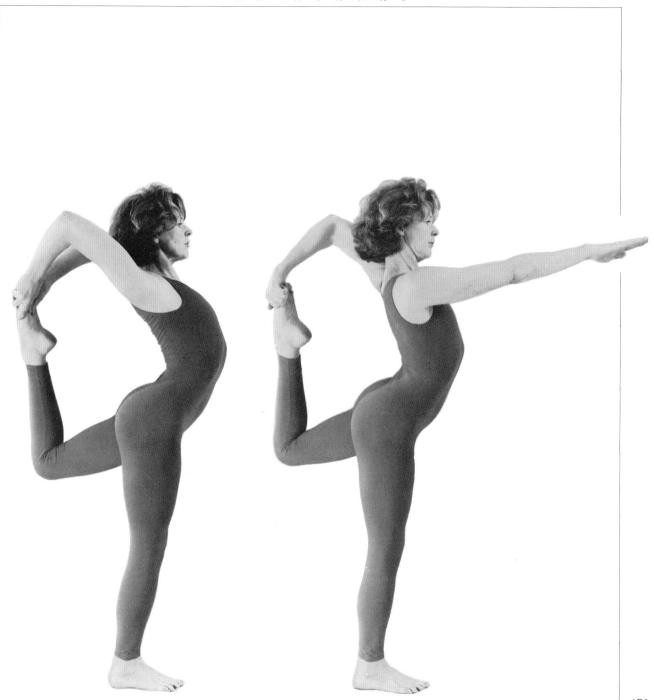

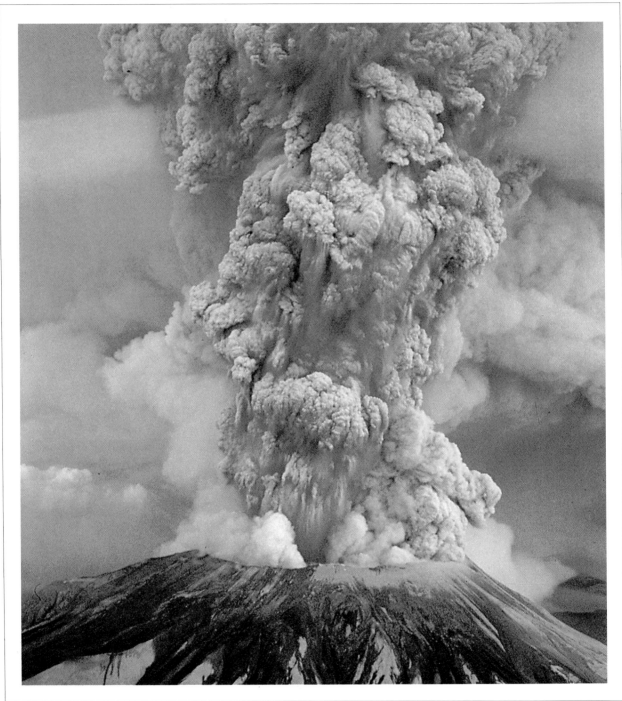

Part III

Breathing

Inhalation – Exhalation – Pranayama.

Breathing

BREATHING IS THE ESSENCE of yoga. Breathe naturally, without forcing. No pressure, no disturbance, nothing should interfere with the simple, tide-like movement of our lungs as we breathe in and out.

After a while, when the last three vertebrae closest to the ground start to receive life, if we are attentive, we will discover that the energy running along the back of the spine (from its base to the top of the head) increases in power, making the spine alive and strong.

Breathing is the most important part of yoga practice. Once we start breathing, training cannot be interrupted, it must be done regularly each day.

We can breathe lying down in Savasana, but the best position is always Padmasana, the cross-legged lotus pose. Should there be difficulty holding this pose, you can sit on your heels (with a strap around the heels to keep them in place). This pose is called Virasana.

Sit comfortably with the spine erect.

Start with "Kapalabhati" and finish with simple breathing, inhaling and exhaling regularly. Some variations can be done in between.

What is important is the regularity of the breathing. Do not try to take long breaths, their length will slowly increase; it is only a question of time.

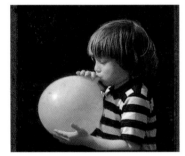

A gaily painted hot air balloon drifting above Tennesee. To maintain such a craft in the sky there needs to be a constant replenishment of hot air gases. Likewise in the body there needs to be a constant cycle of renewal and yet we take for granted this almost unconscious life-giver. Yoga can bring a conscious attention to this ever renewing source.

* Padmāsana is the pose in which you sit with legs crossed. Sit on the ground, bend one knee and put your foot over the thigh; bring the other leg equally crossed over the other thigh. Keep both knees on the floor, the head erect with the chin slightly pulled inside, towards the neck. The moment the weight of the body drops on the earth, the spine elongates and becomes straight.

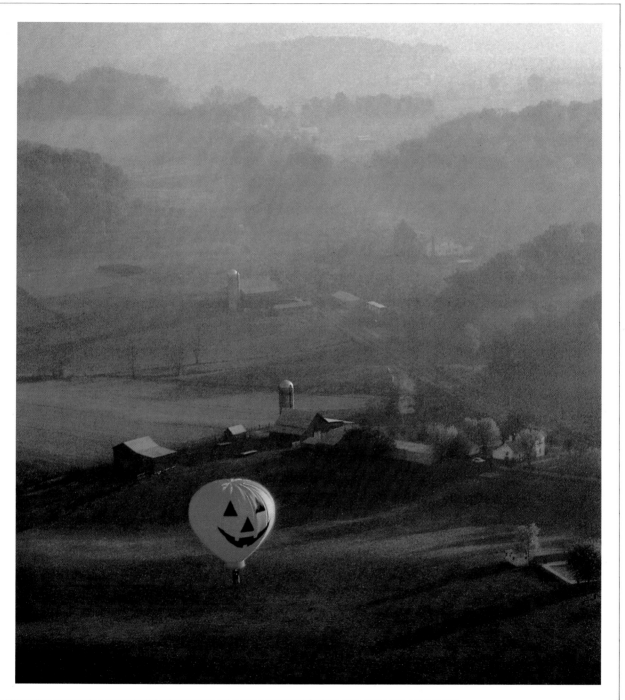

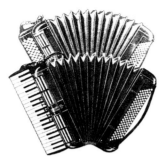

Inhalation

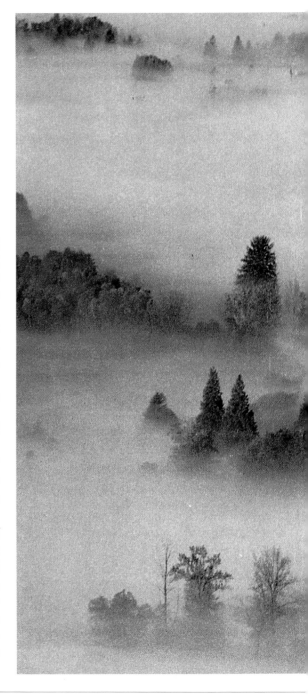

N O BENEFIT IS TO BE GAINED from forcing the breath. To inhale without pushing the air into the lungs and to exhale without wanting to push the air out is rarely done in a happy and easy way.

Do not be tense when you inhale. Do not get involved, but receive the air in a passive, detached way, as though you were only an observer, an outsider.

After exhalation, new air replaces that which has been pressed out, slowly filling the lungs again. There is beauty in this non-action and in this state of observation.

The movement of inhalation is an "un-doing" movement in which tension is released. The body must be relaxed so that the lungs can receive the new inflow of air.

These images can help us to follow the wave of inhalation. It is like a balloon swelling gradually as it fills with air, slowly expanding, or a door pushed gently by the wind, or one can compare it to the effect of a slow-motion film. Or, it is like the air pressed out of an accordion and rhythmically drawn in again, having been pressed first, it is now slowly filling once more. Or like an organ's pedal gradually swelling the sound until it fills the whole church.

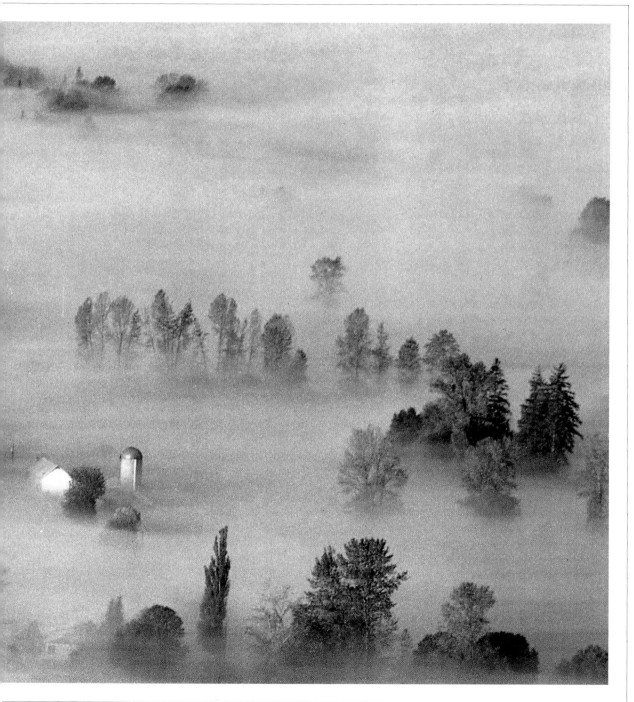

Exhalation

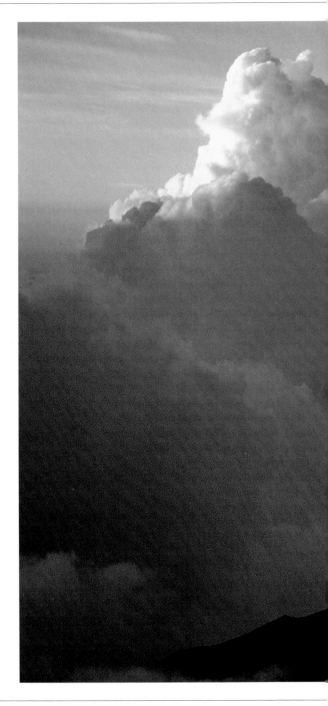

To EXHALE MEANS TO EMPTY the lungs, expelling the air that has been used. The deeper we exhale, the greater is our capacity to inhale new, fresh air. By dropping the hips down (with the lower part of the spine), the body relaxes, making the lungs lighter. This, in turn, enables the bad air (which seeps into the alveoli of the lungs) to be expelled more easily, even from their deeper level.

To exhale correctly, one must begin by allowing the weight of the body to sink towards the ground. It is also helpful to imagine the eyes set at the back of the head, in line with the cerebellum (as described in the section "Reversing") even during inhalation.

There are various images that can be called to mind as one exhales. For instance, let the air rise from deep down the bottom of the spine, towards the top of the head, like a volcano in eruption where the double pull (formed by the pressure of "mass-energy" = gravity, existing at the center of the earth since the beginning of time) releases the lava from the volcano's crater.

Or, if you prefer, picture a flower on the solar plexus opening its petals one after the other until the flower is completely exposed.

Or a fountain of water surging upwards, pushed from the base by a strong jet and coming down in a wide circle.

Or a tree spreading its branches wide and upwards at the same time.

The important thing is that the outflowing breath should expand in a large wave.

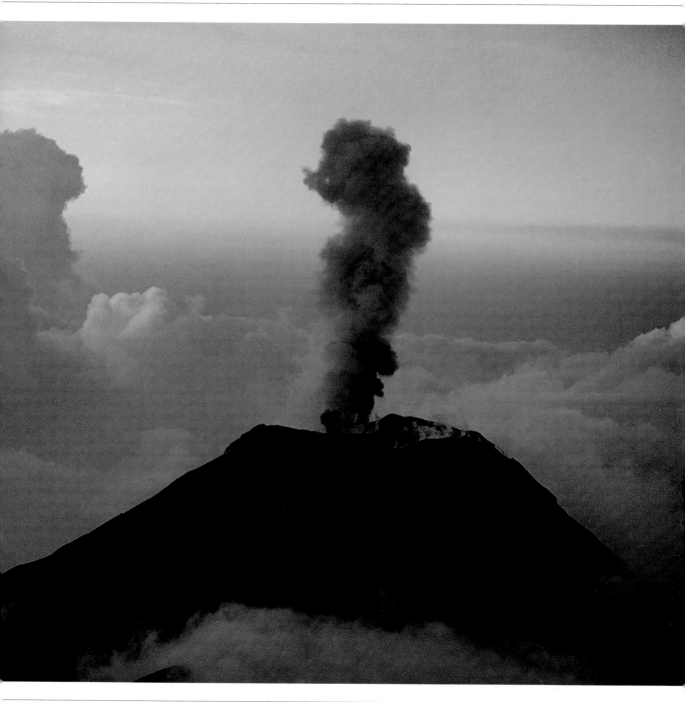

Pranayama

SOME OF THE WELL-KNOWN VARIATIONS of "Pranayama" are listed here
to illustrate the benefits obtained by the body during breathing
practice.

Kapālabhāti

As you exhale you can feel the spine elongating in two opposite
directions, dividing the body in two opposite parts.

Nādī (breathing from alternate nostrils)

Nādī implies breathing only with one nostril at a time. With the
point of your finger press against that little bone that sticks out in the
middle of the nose in order to interrupt the passage of air from that
side, and breath through the other nostril.

Inhale from one nostril and exhale from the other; inhale from
the same nostril and exhale from the other; inhale from the same
one and exhale from the other, and so on and on.

To block the passage of air, use the thumb and the fourth finger,
bending the other finger slightly against the palm of the hand.

This frees the forehead from pressure and strain and makes
headaches disappear.

Retention

While retaining the air after inhalation (when the lungs are full of
air), do not hold the lungs in tension. On the contrary, relax the other
parts of your body by dropping the weight into the ground below and
send the air all about the lungs.

When holding after exhalation (when the lungs are empty) the
abdominal muscles are drawn together pushed inside towards the
back, forming a hollow. One feels as though the front and the back
skin of the abdomen almost touch.

It is important not to hold for a long time when the lungs are
empty, as this can be dangerous.

By relaxing the base of the spine, the feeling of gravity increases
and the upper part of the lungs can expand and broaden.

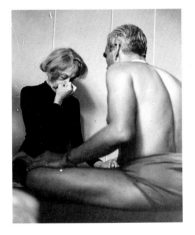

Above: Ivengar teaching the
author Nādī. *Opposite*: Iyengar
exercising Sitali and the "Lion"
pose.

Sītalī

Stretching the tongue forward is of the greatest importance: the tongue increases in length and its edges are strengthened. This improves the throat muscles making speech more articulate, while the thyroid and other glands (such as the parathyroid) will also benefit.

While inhaling, extend the tip of your tongue, throwing it out completely and curling its edges. This will form a small channel in the tongue from which the saliva will be sucked little by little while inhaling. Gradually throw your head back until your ears touch the base of the skull.

Now roll your tongue inside as if you wanted to swallow it. Bring your head down towards the chest, tucking the chin well in and after a few seconds of retention, exhale, keeping your head down. Then push your tongue out anew and start again to inhale.

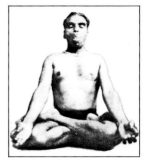

The "lion" pose.

In the lion pose the mouth opens completely and the tongue is exposed in all its length and breadth. It also gives the throat and the lower part of the neck, which cannot otherwise be actively involved, the chance to open.

Inhale with your mouth closed. Exhale with your mouth wide open, throwing your tongue totally out and spreading it in all its width by unfolding the edges and, at the same time, pushing it out and down, as if you wanted to touch the chin with it.

You will feel the extension in your muscles, not only along your throat and neck, but even behind your ears, in the same way as when you yawn.

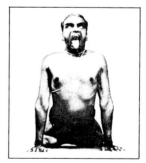

When you have finished your breathing exercises lie down in "Savāsana",* even if only for a few minutes, completely relaxed, breathing naturally and abandoning your body totally to the earth. Do not try to think or meditate but slow down your thoughts. When something comes into your mind, try to increase the space of emptiness between one thought and another.

"Savāsana is silence of the body and the mind".

* Savāsana means to lie supine on the floor with both legs stretched and close to each other, arms extended along the hips, and hands on the ground with palms down. The body in contact with the soil becomes more and more rested and, if you let your head roll once or twice from right to left and from left to right very, very slowly, you will start to relax.

Biography

Vanda Scaravelli was born in Florence on the 15th of January 1908.

She comes from an intellectual and artistic background. Her father, Alberto Passigli, created the "Maggio Musicale Fiorentino", having before formed the "Società degli Amici della Musica" and the "Orchestra Stabile" as he wanted Florence to have its own orchestra.

She was raised in a musical atmosphere surrounded by artists who visited her father's villa "Il Leccio"; Bronislaw Hubermann, Arthur Schabel, Pablo Casals, Adolf Bush, Herman Serkin, Arturo Toscanini, Andres Segovia and others were often guests of the family. Pupil of Ernesto Consolo, Signora Scaravelli has a degree of piano from the Conservatorio Luigi Cherubini in Florence.

She also took part in one of the courses that the well-known conductor, Hermann Scherchen, was then teaching in Paris for orchestra directing. She is still engaged with music, has contact with musicians and many young students who consult her for advice.

Her mother, Clara Corsi, graduated in pedagogy and was among the first Italian women to attend university. She was also a good pianist and studied with a pupil of the famous Antoine Rubinstein.

Her brother, Franco Passigli, was the director of the E.I.A.R. (Radio Television) in Florence. After the death of his father, he took on the presidency of the "Società degli Amici della Musica" in Florence. He was also asked to work in New York for the U.N.'s cultural department where he remained for several years.

Her husband, Luigi Scaravelli, was a professor of philosophy and taught at the universities of Pisa and Rome. He was a very prominent scholar and published several books including "Kant and Modern Physics", "The Critic of Understanding"; some of his books became text-books and are still used today by university students.

Signora Scaravelli lives in a villa on a farm outside Fiesole, among the hills of Florence surrounded by cypresses and olive trees cultivated organically.

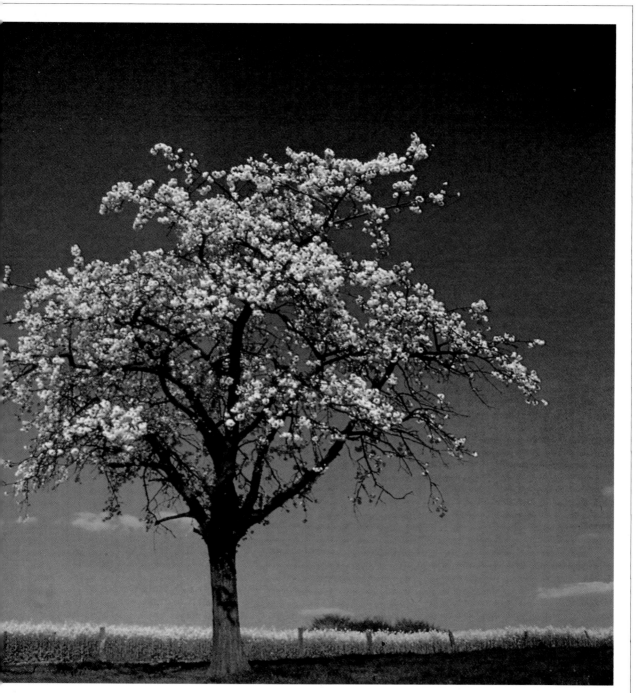

Her house has always been a center where artists and scientists from all over the world met. Among the guests have been included Bernard Berenson, Wolfgang Pauli, Benedetto Croce, Aldous Huxley, Frédéric Leboyer, Buckminster Fuller, Federico Fellini, Jacques Copeau and Terence Stamp.

Her musician friends liked to play for her and even gave concerts in the music room where, in the silence of the night, one could hear a nightingale's voice between Mozart's and Beethoven's notes.

A bust of Signora Scaravelli, sculpted by Libero Andreotti, can be seen in the Modern Art Gallery of Palazzo Pitti in Florence.

Now she is mostly dedicated to help teachers and students through a serious but enjoyable approach in the various yoga exercises bringing the spine back to its original suppleness and readjusting the body, that for so long has been neglected, to regain its strength, health and youth.

Her new teaching is an experience that has transformed many bodies and lives.

Acknowledgements

The publishers and the authors wish to thank the following for allowing reproduction of their photographs and drawings in the present work: B.K.S. Iyengar, Pupul Jayakar and Dona Holleman.

Science Photo Library, London: 23, 56, 102, 122. ZEFA Photo Library, London: 29, 35, 82, 116, 117, 134. Susan Griggs, London: 11, 40, 43, 75, 113, 174, 181. Pictor International, London: 103. Bridgeman Art Library: 89, 102, 118. Image House Photo Library, London: 8/9, 62. Vanda Scaravelli: 2, 7, 8, 20/21, 22/23, 24, 28, 36, 38, 41, 50, 53, 54, 58, 65, 66, 73, 74, 88, 106, 151, 169, 182. Arturo Patten: 143, 145, 147, 148/149, 150, 152, 154/155, 157, 160/161, 164/165, 170/171, 172/173. Dona Holleman, (hand-drawn figurines): 138/139, 142, 144, 146, 148/149, 150/151, 153, 155, 156, 159, 162/163, 165, 167, 168, 170. Lennart Nilson: 18. Studio Reichelt: 60/61. B.K.S. Iyengar: 19, 168, 183. Pupul Jayakar: 27, 45. Labyrinth Picture Library:12/13, 14, 16/17, 26, 30/31, 33, 34, 37, 39, 44, 46/47, 48/49, 51, 57, 59, 63, 64, 67, 70/71, 72, 79, 80/81, 82, 84/85, 86, 90/91, 92, 98/99, 100/101, 106, 108/109, 110/111, 123, 124/125, 129, 130, 135, 137, 140, 158, 176/177, 178/179. Rohit Chawla: 96. Leonardo Da Vinci: 50, 94/95, 118/119. Henri Rousseau: 32. Paul Martin: 52. Herbert List: 55. Frederic Weiss: 68. Harry Wilks: 76. Irving Penn: 77. Saul Steinberg: 115. Sw. Premgit, Devon: 93, 112, 120, 126/127, 128, 131, 132/133.

References

(1) O.J. Ressel, "*Disc Regeneration: Reversibility is possible in Spinal Osteoarthritis*", International Review of Chiropractical, March/April 1989.

(2) Althea Braithwaite, "*How my Body Works*", Dinosaur Publications.

(3) Translated from the Italian, "*Colonna Vertebrale e salute*", Istituto Nazionale "Static", Via Domodossola 9A, Milano.

(4) Joseph Heller and William A. Henkin, "*Body Wise. Regaining your natural flexibility and vitality for maximum well-being*", Jeremy P. Tarcher Inc., Los Angeles, p.23.

(5) Deepak Chopra M.D., "*Quantum Healing. Exploring the Frontiers of Mind Body Medicine*", Bantam Books, New York, p.95.

(6) Ibid., p.99.

(7) Paul Diel, "*Le Symbolisme dans la Mithologie Greque*", Ed. Payit Petite Biblioteque Payot 7, p.150 (Freely translated from French).

(8) Ibid.

(9) J. Krishnamurti.

(10) From the Bible: I Corinthians 15.53.

(11) Paul Diel, "*Symbolism in Greek Mythology*", Shambala, Boulder and London, 1980.

(12) From the Bible.

(13) Paul Diel, "*Symbolism in Greek Mythology*", Shambala, Boulder and London, 1980, p.125.

(14) Joseph Heller and William A. Henkin, "*Body Wise. Regaining your natural flexibility and vitality for maximum well-being.*" Jeremy P. Tarcher Inc., Los Angeles, p.27.

(15) From "*Medicine. An Illustrated History*" by Albert S. Lyons M.D. and R. Joseph Petruccelli,II, M.D., Abradale Press, Harry Abrams Inc., New York, p.187.

(16) Hermann Hesse, "*Siddhartha*".

(17) From "*The Complete Works of Chuang Tzu*", tr. by Burton Watson, Columbia University Press, New York, 1968, pages 77-78.

(18) Kunio Miura, "*The Revival of Qui. Taoist Meditation and Longevity Techniques*". Edited by Livia Kohd. The Univeristy of Michigan, Center for Chinese Studies, 1989, p.338.

(19) Ibid. p.339.

(20) Ibid. p. 253.

(21) Catherine Despeau, "*Gymnastic. The Ancient Tradition. Taoist Meditation and Longevity Techniques*". Edited by Livia Kohd, The University of Michigan, Center for Chinese Studies, Vol.69, 1989.

(22) J. Krishnamurti, "*Education and the Significance of Life*", Introduction, translated freely from Italian "*L'Educazione e il significato della vita*", Ed. La Nuova Italia, Dcc. 1958, pag. V.

(23) John Boslough, "*Searching the Secrets of Gravity*", p. 563.

(24) National Geographic Magazine, May 1989, Vol. 175, p.57

(25) F.J. Bueche, "*Understanding the World of Physics*", McGraw-Hill, 1981, translated from the Italian "*Capire la Fisica*", Ed. Principato.

(26) Elisabeth Ripely, "*Leonardo da Vinci. A Biography*", Henry Z. Walck, University Press, 1900(?), p.48.

(27) Ibid., p.50.

(28) Ibid.

(29) Gary Zukav, "*The Dancing Wu Li Masters. An Overview of the New Physics*", Ed. Fontana Collins, p.41.

(30) Translated from Italian "*Lo Zen*" by W. Watts, a cura di Umberto Eco, Ed. Bompiani, p.100. Original title: "*The spirit of Zen*".

(31) Isabelle Robinet, "*Taoist Meditation and Longevity Techniques*". Edited by Livia Kohd, The University of Michigan, Center for Chinese Studies, Vol. 61, p. 190.

(32) "*La Divina Commedia di Dante Alighieri con il commento di Tommaso Casini*", Sesta edizione rinnovata e accresciuta per cura di S.A. Barbi, Volume unico, G.S. Sansoni Editore, Firenze, p.1067, verso 144.

Index